Do Cheese Puffs Grow on Trees?

Your Health, Your Body, Your Life

Book I

Dr. Dani Torchia, PhD

Dear Amanda, Much love + health Dr Dani Torchia PhD 2021

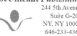

DocUmeant *Publishing*
244 5th Avenue
Suite G-200
NY, NY 10001
646-233-4366
www.DocUmeantPublishing.com

DO CHEESE PUFFS GROW ON TREES?: *Your Health, Your Body, Your Life*
Book 1
Mariana Daniela Torchia, MPH, ACE, R.D., Ph.D.

Published by
DocUmeant Publishing
244 5th Avenue, Suite G-200
NY, NY 10001
646-233-4366

Editors: Serena Tarica www.SerenaTarica.com and Philip S. Marks

Cover Design by Patti Knoles, www.virtualgraphicartsdepartment.com

Back Cover Illustration by Tom Vicini www.drawingfool.com

Illustrations by Vincent Yee www.VincentYeeStudio.com

Additional Illustrations by Lindy Plunkett

Layout by DocUmeant Designs www.DocUmeantDesigns.com

Library of Congress Number: 2021930869

ISBN#: 978-1-950075-36-2 (pbk)
ISBN#: 978-1-950075-37-9 (ePub)
ASIN: B08V6ST3H7

DEDICATION

For all those people whose journey has led them to this book. There are no accidents.

Thank you, Tony, for being a beautiful gift and miracle. You make so many miracles possible.

Contents

ACKNOWLEDGMENTS

Thank you to all those who contributed to reading, editing, supporting, and encouraging the process of book publishing.

I share a special thank you to my first eyes on the first edit, Serena Tarica, and to the final edits through DocUmeant Publishing. The support of my friends, and family has kept me focused, and inspired. Thank you to all those who will read and share the pages of this book, and who will indulge in all the new pages to come.

To the journey!

INTRODUCTION

YOUR MINDSET, PHYSIOLOGY, spirit, knowledge about food and emotional motivators line the pathway to your happiness and health and all contribute to *Do Cheese Puffs Grow on Trees? Your Health, Your Body, Your Life*. This book is designed to help you understand how your health and mind-set work together and how knowledge and insight about foods, your mind and body can help you make choices that improve your whole experience in life. A joyful life of eating for health and eating for enjoyment without guilt is freeing. This is your personal journey into your fabulous health. Scientific data and my experience and knowledge will help me chart my course as your personal cheerleader and teacher. Your health journey is in your hands too. Individual chemical and genetic makeups, appetites, food sensitivities and the intricacies of digestion play a huge part in health, "cravings" and enjoyment of food and life. As you are inspired, you will create your individual path designed around your personality, personal taste, physiology and lifestyle needs. The goal is to find your health and happiness by understanding your mind, your body, the wild world in your tummy and how your "brain tummy" and mind all work together so you can find the best path to a great and healthy life. It's all about **YOU** this time.

Over the past twenty-two years, I have worked in the field of public health and nutrition counseling clients and patients from all walks of life and circumstances: from people in wheelchairs to competitive athletes . . . those who have fallen on hard times and visited food banks, to clients who have had private chefs! I've counseled single working mothers, abused women and children, privileged children, musicians, actors . . . even stressed-out corporate executives and menopausal women who couldn't seem to rid themselves of the tire around their waist and new mothers who gained stubborn baby fat of their own. Even a young man who wanted to gain muscle mass to impress a lucky cutie pie had sought an appointment! I was privileged to be part of a non-profit community clinic in Southern California, where I saw 1,000s of patients over the 21-½ years as a proud interdisciplinary clinician at Valley Community Healthcare (VCH). Each patient whom I counseled on nutrition and health both at VCH and through my private practice sought out personalized guidance to find that sweet spot of self-awareness, self-care, and nutritional know-how in order to live an optimum life with an extraordinary lifestyle.

My focus today is to help anyone who wishes to make a difference in their health, from the hard-working mom, to the corporate jetsetter, all of whom rarely make time for themselves . . . who get up early, work all day, either have 5 a.m. conference calls, or clean and cook endlessly when they get home, who then help someone else in their family or friends and barely get any sleep before they start the whole routine all over again the next day. So many people are in survival mode. The "rat race" is true for all walks of life; but most people I see do not even consider the importance of treating their bodies as well as they treat their cars!

Who am I? Like many of you, my study and career path were presented to me based on my own personal struggle with health and the desire to heal myself and others. I ventured into academia to help heal the world! Science called. I delved into a double-Master's program in clinical nutrition and biochemistry and in public health promotion and education, with a minor in exercise physiology. It was grueling and amazing and since it was a double degree, I had double of everything: Theses, oral presentation, exams, research and internships, the national nutrition exam—insane and magical all at once. I imagined getting my Doctorate right after graduation, but life and work got in the way and it wasn't until much later that I took the PhD plunge. Thank God, as that has changed my life and fulfilled a lifelong expectation that I had since I was 12 years old. The only difference was that at age 12 I imagined being a psychologist, which I quickly realized after graduating with a B.A. in Psychology, was not for me as my initial internship in counseling and therapy made it clear that I was way too animated, interactive and hyper to pull off that career. I had spent all my childhood and young woman years dancing, performing, creatively expressing myself with movement and speaking with those wild Italian hand gestures—a completely different spirit energy in me—so instead, interactive health and sciences with the ability to present to others were all together perfect for my animated personality. *It* was a worthy sacrifice to complete the dissertation and receive the PhD in Public Health and with my nutrition science backilogramsround they both have blended themselves into a perfect delicious dish to do what I absolutely love: help others be empowered through health.

When it comes to implementing your own Nutrition Plan the first thing you need to consider is what is *true* for you. What level of energy feels right? What are your sleep patterns? Could they be improved? What is your body type and ideal body weight for health (not skinniness)? I will be part of your motivational team to help you have fun in life again through great guiltless food, empowering thoughts and an inspiring lifestyle! Together, we will make new discoveries about your health and well-being. I will provide you with resources and tips which I have seen make a positive difference to countless people, including myself. To help you *avoid* having to read hundreds of peer-reviewed publications presented by experts in their fields, the plethora of experienced doctors, registered dietitians, nurse practitioners, statisticians, health experts and Ph.D.'s, I combined my experience and theirs in *Do Cheese Puffs Grow on Trees?: Your Health, Your Body, Your Life* to help make life *easier* for you and save you from the virtual impossibility of locating, gaining access to ($$), reading and understanding the current relevant scientific research. You can always look the research up as I provide references for you.

THIS IS NOT A DIET BOOK!

Diets (dieting, deprivation) do not work long term and they are not realistic as a lasting lifestyle for eating. So, which things do work for the long term? Having the complete and fabulous awareness of who you are, what's making you "tick" and recognizing your own relationship to food are all important. Food is necessary for survival, so learning to have a satisfying, healthy relationship with food is essential to your success. There are many extreme ways to lose weight, including fad liquid diets, liposuction, stomach stapling, plus the traditional method—starvation. It might be good to avoid short-term, painful, food-deprivation extreme diet choices. Instead, embark on a journey of self-discovery and knowledge about food and energy that are easy to process. If surgery is necessary, that's okay too, but six months of self-care and nutrition counseling is encouraged first! Gentler more lasting approaches include understanding the physiology between your brain and your gut, recognizing chemical and food reactions, as well participating in group support with like-minded people/ friends and licensed therapists, nutrition experts and counselors.

For some, opening up to spiritual perspectives has been transforming. An inclusive approach to your body and mind awareness, combined with information about what works long-term, will create a successful and exciting new path to Inspire Your Health for life!

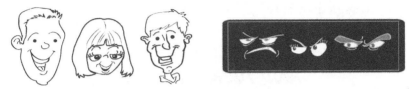

Keep the Happy Folks and Avoid the Grumpy Heads

Be with happy and like-minded people. Grumpy people who hang around other grumpy people have a hard time making the leap to happiness. Forget those critical grumpy heads and find your joy.

What's in this book?

Conflicting dietary guidelines can make a person give up on reading about health. Two bottom lines are: "Is what you're eating working for you?" *and* "Can you keep on going." What is tasty and keeps you healthy? What does the long-term research say? Do what makes sense and works for you. It doesn't matter what trending book you read . . . utilize scientific data that demonstrates longevity and health as it incorporates the things that make sense in your life, values, lifestyle and beliefs. If you don't feel well, find the way to renewed energy. Just because something seemed good for *Joe Schmo* doesn't mean it's right for you.

Be honest with yourself and, by all means *enjoy* the process of discovery! Think of new and exciting changes as *lifestyle choices* that provide health and joy, rather than resorting to extreme makeover tactics or temporary deprivation diets. Life is full of twists and turns, stressors and gifts. Choose Your Health, Your Body and Your LIFE! Just like the book's title. Choose what helps you enjoy health and life to its fullest, no matter your circumstances. Surround yourself with kind, encouraging, helpful, health-minded people. Your surroundings matter, choose kind people and be kind. Choose laughter and laugh. Enjoy your life! No matter the hardships, look up, follow the lead of those who have struggled and keep going no matter what.

THE PSYCHOLOGY OF EATING AND YOUR MIND SET

What is YOUR SECRET to HEALTH?

There is and has been *a lot* of "hoopla" regarding fabulous, yet at times, confusing weight-and-health data! When it comes to health, learning how to navigate your nutritional choices is the first step toward your lifelong goal. I want to share my 23 plus years of clinical and life-experience so you will be inspired to believe in yourself and have the belief that you will reach your health goals. I have put together tips and tools on food and body while never emphasizing going on a diet. Most of us know that the whole diet cycle is more of a "Hamster-wheel" experience, that leaves many disillusioned and unmotivated.

> **Be healthy, happy, and free to be . . . no matter what your circumstances.**
>
> Your first step is your first step.
>
> Your beginning is perfect for your unique circumstances.
>
> Listen to those whom you admire and respect.
>
> Those who have come from your circumstances and experiences and are experiencing life the way you want to experience life
>
> (not materialism, but their essence of happiness, joy, and sparkle) are perfect motivators.

Instead, all these pages are meant for YOU: This is about you. This book reminds you to listen to your body and to pay attention to the changes that work for you and be okay with those that don't.

Having energy is a great motivator to help your body and soul feel free and to help you continue to do the things that inspire *you*: Youthful, Optimistic and Unstoppable. It may sound corny, but it's true. Why not imagine the best for *yourself*? The greatest motivator is having energy. With energy, you feel fantastic. When you feel energized, you are able to do things in life that inspire you and keep you motivated. One activity builds the next...every step you take toward health-minded lifestyle choices and *activates* your desire to keep doing the things that inspire more well-being.

CHEESE PUFFS DON'T GROW ON TREES . . . OR DO THEY?

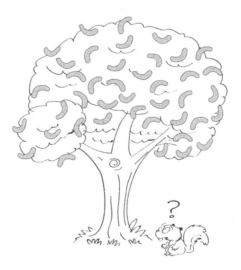

Why did I decide to write this book series? Let's take a trip back in time to that turning point! It was a typical Southern California morning and I was ready to joyfully tackle the day's sessions at the Southern California community clinic where over 18 years of my life had been dedicated as a clinical nutritionist and where I was working throughout my PhD program. When I looked at my schedule, every appointment from 10 a.m. to 5 p.m. on the Electronic Health Record was booked: I saw my list of 13 patient names. I gulped down my green tea, took a deep breath and started. Hours passed as I educated a mix of hesitant, disbelieving and eager patients on health goals, reviewed lab results and doctor's recommendations to inspire them for long-term success. I felt good, yet there was an air of something about to happen—I just didn't know that it was going to be a creative and life altering moment!

It was 2:00 p.m. when my book-inspiring patient arrived. We will call her Rose. She was a menopausal woman struggling with her weight at nearly 280 pounds. She was missing most of her front teeth due to life's tribulations and this high-school graduate had come to depend on her daughter for financial support and so ended up at her non-profit community health center.

"Hello, welcome! How can I help you today?" I asked.

Rose replied timidly, "I guess my doctor sent me to you because of my weight . . ." I asked if she was ready to look at new choices and Rose nodded yes. I proceeded with a 24-hour Food Recall and Monthly Food Intake Review, reviewed her labs and medical chart record with her. I listened as Rose shared information about her lifestyle and described typical daily meals. Rose's blood labs showed that something she was doing was not working for her, as the fat and cholesterol in the blood were too high and her poor liver was saying "cut it out" based on the high concentration of liver enzymes we measured (high liver enzymes can mean inflammation and fatty liver disease). Basically, her blood sugar, cholesterol and fat (triglycerides) were high and so were her *liver* markers. In her case, the high sugar intake and processed fats contributed not only to the out-of-range lab values, but also to her low energy level and weight gain.

It might look like a "That's terrible!" moment, but this is and has been extremely common in my practice. Nearly 75% of the patients, both in the community clinic and in private contracts, have had similar health issues. Rose and I spent the next thirty minutes discussing her food choices. To make life easier for her, I played "make a healthy plate" with my life size rubber food models as we put together potential meal and snack selections for her to try. She was surprised at how much food a person was "allowed" to eat when the food was considered whole (not processed) and fresh. At the end of our session I asked a question, as I always do, to make sure she was comfortable with what to do on her own. "Now that we've gone through all the foods, what are some good snack choices that you would like to try?" Without missing a beat Rose replied, "How about CHEETOS®? I really like CHEETOS. Can I eat those as snacks?" I took a breath to avoid responding inappropriately, so I replied in a kind and gentle voice, "It's good to ask yourself this question whenever you are not sure if something is healthy or not . . . in this case."

"Do CHEETOS come from the Earth, a tree, or a factory?"

I waited a few seconds . . . keeping my eyes gently focused on her as I awaited her response. She took a deep breath and responded, "I don't know?" After almost two decades of having seen hundreds of patients, day-in and day-out, I certainly had not expected that response.

So, I'd like to share with you the correct answer: **Cheese Puffs don't grow on trees. . . .**

. . . They are made in a factory with processed chemicals and offer zero nutritional value, though some would argue the cheddar cheese is worthy; I can hear you! However, they do taste good

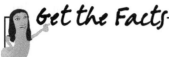 **Get the Facts**

Ten Working Tips

1. EAT when you're hungry (more on this "feedback loop" of why you're hungry) within a set period of time; take some hours off without eating to help clean those cells, burn stored fat, and regenerate cells.
2. CHOOSE nutrient-rich foods that keep you energized.
3. BALANCE is what matters. NEVER deprive yourself—trust your common sense.
4. LEARN what works for your body.
5. REST, SLEEP, MEDITATE, ACCEPT, FORGIVE, BREATHE!
6. PAY ATTENTION to food cues: emotional, spiritual, environmental.
7. ENJOY and forget the guilt!
8. RESEARCH, and CHOOSE.
9. Find a buddy.
10. Give it 7 days and keep counting . . . start with 24 hours and keep going.

and are part of our nation's processed food frenzy; often a daily staple, as I've witnessed at the clinic, school lunch yards and most convenience stores.

Rose totally threw me off my calm self-mode that day. As soon as I was finished with her appointment, I marched straight into the Medical Director's office, sat on the worn-out chair next to his desk, sighed as he interrupted, "What is going on? You look . . ." (He probably wanted to say 'crazed'.) I looked up at him and spurted out, "I have no idea what I am doing here today. I just spent 30 minutes teaching and after all that . . . not a healthy food option was selected by her, but instead she thought CHEETOS grew on trees! I think I am doing this all wrong?"

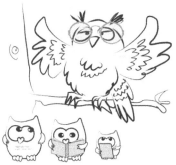

He laughed and said, "I think you are burnt out and should take some time off, I will authorize the leave, as you have vacation time, I am sure, after all those years you've worked here." I must have looked like a crazy person for the Medical Director to say, "Go home, don't worry about it, take a mental health break." I thought to myself, "Now, I have to put things into perspective." I, along with the dedicated clinicians there, nurses, nurse practitioners and medical doctors, spend intense time with less than 20 minutes per high-risk patient 40 or more hours per week, with very difficult patients and at times limited resources not only for us but for them. After 18 or more years of doing something repeatedly, there is a risk of burn out, or a sense of, "is anything I am doing working?" However, even with wild work frustration and occasional feelings of hopelessness . . . OF COURSE it matters what I did, what I do and what anyone else does, but sometimes, a little break in the pattern can lead to amazing new things. Our dear Rose was my angel; through my frustration that day, she inadvertently led me to writing, researching and learning more on how to help others in even better and more effective ways.

After this awakening encounter with my patient, I decided to write a book about nutrition for the hard-working person who just hasn't gotten a break, or who wishes to know more to envision and achieve a healthy future. Many years as a clinical nutritionist inspired me to help people reach their health goals and be confident and aware of the surprising simplicity of eating well for life. Thank goodness, it is easier than you might think—you just have to "get yourself" and believe. Great things do grow on trees and are accessible to you! . . . That's what we all need to eat. Foods that grow on a tree or come from the earth are the staples of good health. Occasional CHEETOS that grow on the famous CHEETOS assembly line are okay, if you must, but keep in mind they may sabotage your goals! There are options.

My confession: In high school I loved stuffing CHEETOS into my tuna sandwich; oh, so tasty!

Let's get started with the Prelude with a Sneak Peek, trivia and cheat sheet list for you

QUICK CHEAT SHEET! WHAT DO I EAT?

Generally Acceptable Healthy Heart and Lifestyle Choices in Scientific Data

- Plant foods rock: 10 servings a day of veggies and fruits keep tons of diseases away (P.S. generally more veggies than fruit due to fructose content of fruit)
- Lean protein: 6 servings or less a day
- Legumes, nuts, seeds: 4–5 servings a week
- Grains (non-GMO or unaltered): 6–8 servings a day (adapt to your needs) make sure you are non-reactive to grains which contain gliadin or gluten
- Dairy: 2–3 servings (vegans or others can sub this)
- Healthy Oils: 1–2 servings a day

What's a Serving?

- Veggies (plant): ½ cup cooked or 1 cup raw leafy greens
- Fruits (plant): ½ cup or ¾ cup of berries—berries have less sugar
- Protein: 3 ounces (3 x 3 x 1 inch) or 1 egg, preferably fish/poultry vs red meats or vegetarian sources
- Unrefined Grains: ½ cup cooked, 1 slice
- Dairy: 8 ounces milk or yogurt, or 1-ounce cheese, ½ cup cottage cheese
- Beans/Legumes: ½ cup cooked (also good as protein for vegetarians)
- Nuts: 1-ounce about 15–20 almonds, or 5–7 walnuts (also good as protein for vegetarians)
- Oils: 1 tablespoon, ¼ avocado, nut oils from nuts

What's a Legume?

- Legumes are plants which produce seed pods. High in lectins (family of proteins hard to break down)—some people react to these. Pay attention to how you feel. All plant foods have some lectins, but some such as legumes are high in lectins.
- Peas, beans, lentils and peanuts—yup, peanuts are not considered nuts.

TRIVIA: LIZARD TAILS AND US!

Lizard tails come back and so do some of our CELLS.

Your tummy lining regenerates every 5–7 days; taste buds change every 10 days; red blood cells regenerate every 4 months; your liver really is like a lizard's tail and can regenerate damaged cells completely within 30 days—that's if what's messing up the liver is no longer there (Tylenol overdose, alcohol, viruses).

We replace about 50–70 billion cells every day!

CANCER RISK REDUCTION STUDIES!

Cancer and Disease studies of 69,120 participants in the Adventist Health Study found:[1]

- Statistically significant reduction in cancer cases for vegetarians and vegans compared to all others

BUT: non-vegetarians who ate >5 servings of vegetables decreased their risk of disease too.

Oxford University study, 2013, analyzed the following:[2]

- This study of 45,000 people found vegetarians had 32% less heart disease, lower blood pressure, lower bad cholesterol and lower weight than non-vegetarians.

PS: Much more on this in later chapters, *this is not a book about being a vegetarian*, but it will emphasize the amazing health benefits of **adding** plant-based foods to your diet.

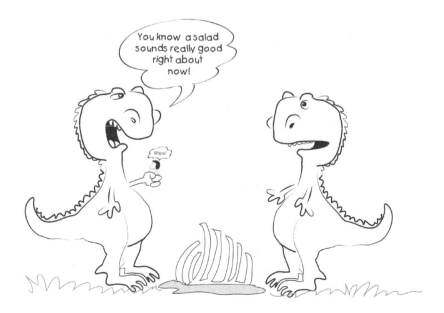

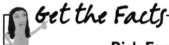

Get the Facts

Risk Factors for
Overweight and Obesity

- Genetics
- Lack of activity
- Stress
- Depression (chicken or the egg)
- Excess eating
- Excessive sugar, beverage, and alcohol consumption
- Environmental pollutants as endocrine disruptors
- Food reactions (pay attention to how you respond to each food)
- Poor quality calories
- Sleep deprivation
- Medications: antidepressants, lithium, steroids, birth control, hormone replacement therapy with estrogen or progesterone . . .
- Illness: polycystic ovarian syndrome (PCOS), pituitary tumors, hypothyroidism or thyroid tumors, autoimmune disorders, etc.
- Eating all the time without enough breaks—over feeding self
- Socioeconomic circumstance
- Mind-set and Belief Systems
- Eating Disorders—binging, purging, dysregulation
- And more—each person will have a different biochemical reaction to medications, hormones, and environmental factors

CHAPTER 1

Easy Breezy Motivation and Purpose!

THE PSYCHOLOGY OF YOUR HEALTH

EVEN THOUGH I will teach you about food and share fun scientific facts about health and nutrition, **I don't want you to be obsessed or worried about what you can and cannot eat.** This book is a guide to find your perfect plan. I will give you examples to increase awareness and motivation. The steps you take are entirely your own. I will give you useful sources of information on current food and health trends. You might be surprised at the incredible increases that have occurred over the years related to how much food is produced and consumed, as well as how many whacky health and weight trends exist; many are helpful, though. I will shed light on chemicals in your food and on which chemicals are banned from country to country. The best part is making you aware and comfortable with the information so that all your choices contribute to your health! The purpose of this book is for you to gain relevant knowledge with the freedom to choose and create a plan to help you feel free to eat well without stress on your journey to your optimal health!

First, I will give you the list of tangible FACTORS that affect your actions and power based on scientific research and your state of mind. These factors will contribute greatly to long-term success in all your goals.

What works when it comes to Navigating Nutrition?

- Believe you can do it!
- Believe you are capable and ready!
- Believe you can maintain what works for you!
- Believe you have a range of good options and choices!
- Believe in *yourself*!

BELIEF IN CHANGE MAKES ALL THE DIFFERENCE

A system of success is effective when you, as a whole person, are considered and when your *thought process* is taken into account. Mere temporary behavioral changes aren't as effective as Cognitive Behavior Changes (CBC) which is part of that "self-talk" or what you tell yourself and believe.[3] For some, Cognitive Behavior Therapy (CBT) (https://psychcentral.com/lib/in-depth -cognitive-behavioral-therapy/) is used to help make behavior changes and it involves short-term goals to help navigate problem solving related to your thinking and behavior. It deals with your attitudes, beliefs, images and thoughts and how these cognitive processes (like a machine in your mind) influence your behavior and emotions. If you see a therapist, this type of intervention is more goal oriented and can take five to ten months, or even less for some, compared to long term psychoanalytical processes, which also has its place. But this is not a psychology book! However, our behavior is INFLUENCED by our thoughts and perceptions and that is why I bring CBC and CBT up! Notice your thoughts: It's awesome to pay attention. REMEMBER adaptability—do what works for you. If it works for you, it's working. If it doesn't, it's not working for you! Keep seeking and find that truth that makes sense and is effective for you.

Belief

The key to optimal health is the power of belief in yourself. If you believe you can make healthful changes and maintain them, you are more likely to make those changes. Even if you remember perfectly common-sense things or you know amazing amounts of health data, *belief* that making healthful choices can make a difference is vital for your success. Truly believing and visualizing that something can change in your health for the better is what will give you the motivation and behavioral changes that contribute to your empowerment.

Your body is unique and incredible. *"My body is unique and incredible"*.

Accepting who you are with your body's unique nuances takes the pressure off-of some weird ideal which confuses you with unrealistic expectation of who you are supposed to be. What matters? It's that amazing feeling of health; it's being able to do activities you love that bring joy and fulfillment to your daily life, which in turn contribute to your happiness and motivation and hope. The new YOU: Youthful, Optimistic and Unstoppable is now ready for a healthy self. You have the freedom to choose. Welcome to your success! Your mind and body are ready for you.

You may have heard the phrase: "You are what you eat," but I would like to ADD, **"You are what you think."** Your thoughts about food are food for thought and thoughts ARE a big deal . . . it does matter what you think; not only about yourself but also about food. What you imagine is what you think, so allow yourself to imagine beautiful things.

What helps maintain your weight and health?

You have so many choices when it comes to nutrition that these all can be confusing. Once you make decisions and are comfortable

with realistic plans, then consistent actions give you great results!
I am excited to share with you what I have seen work with my
clients and patients for over two decades. The following are scientifically supported, successful actions that provide excellent
long-term health and weight maintenance: First the list, then the
explanation!

Self-Monitoring and the Cognitive Behavior Theory

Components of What Works
- Self-Efficacy—Social Cognitive Theory
- Goal Setting
- Group Counseling or Group Support
- Behavioral Substitution
- Stimulus Control
- Energy Intake (Calories and Macronutrients)
- Physical Activity and Exercise
- Sleep
- Delicious Nutritious Food

SELF-MONITORING AND COGNITIVE BEHAVIORAL APPROACHES

Self-Monitoring is an excellent tool to start a new process! It
serves as a springboard to build a new routine and increase awareness. It is simply keeping track, in whichever way you like, of
what you eat, how much you exercise and how you feel. This may
include monitoring the time and amount you eat, counting calories (calorie type [what kind of food not just calories] is more
important and counting may not be for you, but it useful as an eye
opener), reviewing how you prepare your meal, rating your hunger, being aware of emotions related to what you want to eat or
when you eat, activities you are performing when you are eating

and weighing yourself. Studies show that self-monitoring provides greater results for longevity of outcomes in weight maintenance and health, than no self-monitoring. There are tons of apps now that help self-monitoring all wellness tracking: calories, fat, vitamins/minerals, exercise, sleep and meditation.

The truth in keeping track of calories consumed is that people generally *underestimate the total calories* and quality of calories they consume by 10 to 30%. That's why frustration sets in and alters the outcome. Self-monitoring provides a vital source of awareness of *actual* calorie consumption and type of calorie consumption, which matter. All forms of self-monitoring result in successful weight loss and maintenance.

Using a pedometer that counts the total steps you take per day is becoming popular, so try it. The minimum number of steps each of us should take every day is 5,000, with a goal of 10,000 (4 miles)! The faster your pace, the more you burn, or the more intense (up-hill) the more you burn ... BUT keep your pace within a steady non exhausting heart rate, otherwise you can defeat the purpose. Good shoes and safety are vital too. Protect your feet and joints.

Those who self-monitor less or not at all frequently have frustrating results or no results compared to those who DO self-monitor.[4]

For example, after 18 weeks of consistent self-monitoring, a group of women lost an average of 33 pounds (15 kilograms), while the non-self-monitors, or those who occasionally self-monitored, lost an average of 9 pounds (4 kilograms).[5] A good reminder to all of us to self-monitor.

Self-monitoring has proven to be extremely successful. Keep in mind that long-term success also occurs when you surround yourself with like-minded people who are on the same journey as you, *no nay-sayers around you*! Healthy dining with family, group support sessions, friends committing to walking together and cheering each other on—all contribute to long-term success. Practice self-monitoring and explore new choices daily!

**Self-monitoring is one aspect of the
Cognitive Behavioral Theory (CBT).**

**Cognitive is your thought process, Behavior
is what you do and Theory is a concept.**

Now is the time to recognize the CUES that trigger your behavior to eat when you are *not* hungry. Awareness changes everything for the good! Once you are aware, your ability to make changes in behavior increases. CBT also asks you to reinforce or reward yourself when you do something that you know is good for you. Rewards can include making special time to see a concert or movie, taking a drive to your favorite place, or going for a nature walk with a friend. Whatever brings you long term gratification supports positive choices.

The good news is that you can learn a new way to react to those triggers, those cues, those "I need to eat more" food cues.

What are food cues? Food cues are based on classical conditioning—you remember a feeling associated with something else . . . the food, smell, or sound can create involuntary responses of salivating, "craving," or wanting something. Food cues can come from what you see, hear, think. or smell. Here is where the billion-dollar *advertisement* budget is so clever! If McDonald's reportedly spent 761 million dollars on advertisement in 2018 and Domino's and Taco bell each spent 415 to 418 million, can you imagine how much money is spent annually on all food advertising?

Advertisers are masters at bringing up those good feelings when you see their logos, or anything else associated with "I want this now." However, it's not only advertisers but anything that can create associations which contribute to eating more. The smell of food can trigger an **involuntary** reaction of salivation, hunger pangs and perceived cravings for that food and so you end up driving somewhere to buy it and eat it, even if you are not hungry in the first place. Most films, TV shows, advertisement posters, billboards and menu art have something placed there *purposefully* to inspire you to eat something or drink something. Your personal associations with music and visual cues create pathways of manipulating your behavior. You can even have food cues that are related to seeing certain people, experiencing certain stress levels, or hearing certain voices. (https://www.psychologytoday.com/us/blog/food-junkie/201301/mind-your-p-s-and-food-cues-0)

Cognitive Behavioral Steps:
1. Goal Directed—measurable results
2. Process Oriented—decide how to make the changes
3. Encourages Small Changes—doable

Self-efficacy: Do you believe you will eat Kale on Fridays?

What is self-efficacy? Self-efficacy is the amount you believe that you *can* do a task or perform a behavior to bring the result you want. It measures *how deeply you believe* you have the power to perform a *specific* behavior such as walking ten minutes or eating kale once a week! This is where the command of thought comes into play. When it comes to health, you need to *believe* you can achieve your goals. Here is an example of how you might measure your level of self-efficacy on a questionnaire:

Question: *On a scale from 1 to 5, how certain am I that I can perform this task?* In other words, *how certain are you that you will exercise at least once a week?*

Answer Options:

1. Not at all
2. Somewhat Uncertain
3. Somewhat Certain
4. Fairly Certain
5. Very Certain

No matter what your goals are, if you are uncertain of your *power* to achieve a result, you are not likely to do it! If you *believe you can*, **you will**!

GOAL SETTING

Most of you have thought about setting goals when it comes to health or weight loss. What stopped you? I have found in my practice that people set extreme and inhuman goals like, "I will lose 50 pounds in 2 months!" Some people thought 50 pounds in 3 weeks was reasonable. For a regular human being who is not a contestant on *The Biggest Loser, or Extreme Make-Over*, losing 50 lbs. in 2 months is a goal that creates frustration and perceptions of failure when the goal is not met. What works? *Small, short-term, measurable and time-tabled goals work.* For example, "I will lose 1–2 pounds a week," which is perfect. You have the power to reach that goal and maintain a healthy weight as you learn about your individual eating cues, emotions, sleep, activity and food intake. Try not to compare your fat loss to others because the more someone needs to lose, the more they are able to lose per week initially as the body re-adjusts to the changes. For some people, five pounds per week is possible, but generally accepted weight loss for most people that maintains LONG-TERM *is one to two pounds per week.* Slow and steady achieves long term success.

What are the Keys to Goal Setting?

1. **Reachable**

    Goals must be attainable and realistic. "Losing four pounds" or "wearing size 16 vs. 18" or "being able to touch my knees vs. thighs as I improve flexibility" or "eating one vegetable cup per day" or "adding one vegetable serving per meal" are doable and real.

2. **Timetable**

    Goals have a set timetable: specified, reasonable deadline such as, "January 15th" or "Monday, July 27th" or "by Sunday". However, they must also have reasonable flexibility to deal with unforeseen circumstances encountered in the real world.

3. **Specified Amount**

    Goals have a realistic and doable quantity such as, "two pounds of weight loss" or "six hours sleep per night vs. four hours" or "losing one-inch around my waist" or "three times per week for 25 minutes."

Keep in mind that rewards should not include money. Research has shown that monetary rewards do not work. You should also not choose a food-related reward as you will only give yourself a psychological cue that says, "If I do well, I can reward myself with food!" Without realizing that rewarding with food creates a "food cue", you might set yourself up to get the munchies when you are hiking. Positive non-food rewards

> **Movies Tickets Not Money!**
>
> Reward yourself for achieving your health, weight, and health goals!

include going to a special performance, taking a hike with a friend, enjoying time you may not normally take on an adventure, or giving yourself a 'special gift' you wouldn't have gotten for yourself otherwise, such as a facial or a massage (not on credit, though). Never go into debt to get a reward. Choose what is easily affordable. You don't want to create a new issue of overspending and creating debt!

Group Support

Social support has a direct influence on your state of being and how well you feel emotionally and physically. Support from others helps you succeed in achieving your dreams and personal goals. *It is important to surround yourself with people who are positive* (not the "friends" that tear you down or insult the people important to you). If you have no choice but to be around negative people, make sure you don't share your intimate dreams and goals with them. They will invariably want to suppress your drive. It is an unfortunate part of human nature, so be aware and love yourself enough to protect your goals so you have the freedom to grow.

Hope and the Combo-Party

For your ultimate success, I want you to know that there is **hope**. You can achieve your health goals. Studies on weight loss and maintenance find excellent long-term results when a comprehensive program, which I call the **Combo-Party** approach, combine social support with stimulus control, self-monitoring and Cognitive Behavioral Theory. Remember, even though food consumption and exercise are important, these are not the only things to consider in your quest for ultimate health. Sometimes, these are not the main culprits, but your *emotional state and your environmental cues* are important contributing factors to consider.

> *In my clinical practice, patients who came to see me one-on-one who also came to my weekly group classes on nutrition and who shared with other participants, had greater long-term success than those who did not come to group classes.*

If you can't be there in person every week, choose an online group or weekly chat with a buddy who is making similar changes. Check out the wonderful online APPS to self-monitor along with group meet-ups for weight loss such as: Weight Watchers, Beach Body™ (online), MyFitness Pal ™ and reach out to community centers and personal coaches who conduct internet and in-person group sessions. You can even start your own health-minded group and meet weekly or even Skype, Facetime, Zoom . . . , or text each other at a set day and time.

Make sure you connect with the group(s) that work for you!

WHAT ELSE COULD YOU DO?

Behavioral Substitution

You are human! Just because you are striving to become conscious about stimulus control, eating cues and so much more doesn't mean you can absolutely eliminate every action that may affect your health adversely. Awareness is a beautiful thing. It is critical to find a desirable alternative behavior. Pay attention to the times that you get cravings or suddenly want to eat—even though you've already eaten. You may just discover a cue! Whether it's eating more than you need or drinking out of stress, it's good to check in with yourself.

IN-LAWS AND BAGELS!

Triggers and Cues

I had a client who noticed that whenever she talked to her in-laws, she suddenly craved bagels with cream cheese along with seven teaspoons of sugar in her coffee! Some call this nervous eating. The underlying emotional causes may not be critical to understand at this point. Identifying triggers is the important activity to begin catching your **CUE**.

Maybe you are stressed in similar situations. If the person makes you uncomfortable, consciously or unconsciously, which causes you to cover that stress with food, it is time to find a **substitute behavior**. Try walking for a few minutes or do relaxation exercises before and after speaking with this person. Substitute the eating behavior with journaling and venting on paper, calling a friend, breathing, or anything you can think of instead of reaching for the fridge. There are many options for you. The great thing is that *you* get to choose which behavioral substitutions you will use! That is your form of *POWER of SELF*. My own behavioral substitutions include hiking, walking around the house, drinking unsweetened green tea or texting my girlfriends to check in; I love using *Whatsapp*. Take a few moments now and make a list of substitution behaviors you would like to try.

- ✓ Substitution Behavior for _____ will be _____ (this is useful for NOT Texting an Ex too!) For example:
- ✓ Substitution behavior for calling X will be to take a walk and call my best friend instead.
- ✓ Substitution behavior for purchasing a box of cookies will be buy one single cookie and eat two **tablespoons** of cottage cheese or nut butter to help with my blood sugar. You can come up with all kinds of alternatives! If there are no cookies (as they can trigger hunger), you can try peaches and cottage cheese, or for a more low-sugar approach, string cheese and carrots, celery and peppers, or hard-boiled egg. Non-dairy approaches with walnuts and raisins. It's your choice as long as it works for you. It can be anything that makes sense to you.

STIMULUS CONTROL OR MAYBE NOT!

The All You Can Eat Restaurant Dilemma!

Every day we are triggered by all kinds of external and internal emotional cues. Good news! We get to recognize what they are and make changes if we want to get positive results.

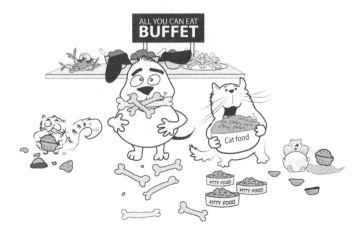

Stimulus control comes from the principle of "conditioning" or what you may know as something that reinforces a behavior. How do you start your day?

Does breakfast happen while you are *rushing to work eating in your car*? If this is you, *you are conditioning your brain to associate eating with the minute you get in your car.* And it's not just your car either, **it's everything you experience while you are driving that can be paired with food trigger habits!**

Do you order a large popcorn and soda whenever you go to the movies? If this is you, you may find that watching a movie *has* to be paired with popcorn and soda because you have trained your brain to eat these foods while doing this particular activity. In this case, watching a movie stirs the craving, or just driving to the movie theatre gets the popcorn salivary glands going! Do you plop down on the couch, turn on the TV and eat dinner after a long day at work? Well, guess what? You are likely to eat anywhere from 25% to 150% more while watching TV, than while NOT distracting yourself with TV. Here is another tidbit: US television networks allow for eight minutes of commercials in 22 minutes of programming; this gives you sixteen minutes of commercials in your one hour "viewing pleasure"! (https://www .quora.com/How-many-commercials-are-in-an-hour-of-tv)

Mindfulness and Eating

This is a good time to practice mindful eating, where you eat and focus only on the food, the texture, the taste and the chewing! *Mindfulness* is paying attention and letting your brain recognize that you are *actually eating* food: Chewing more and noticing the food and texture are the first steps in mindful eating, which will contribute to improved digestion and feeling full.

There are about 11 food commercials per hour on primetime television! Being aware of this helps you recognize *why* you get the munchies while you are watching TV. I started counting how many commercials about foods were shown during my favorite night-time drama. There were three to seven. I did not get 11, however, 11 is reported by Harvard University.[6] I also noticed I wanted to eat more during TV night than during hiking day! We all get to be aware of how we are being manipulated. Awareness is a wonderful tool.

What is an example of positive Stimulus Control?

Positive-stimulus-controls include eating a healthy, satisfying meal at the table *without* the TV, but with good conversation or awareness of the day. You associate eating breakfast, lunch, or dinner with sitting at the table mindfully enjoying healthy food. Mindful means allowing your body to know it is eating without being mentally and physically numbed by TV watching while eating. You might even have wonderful interactive communication with your spouse, kids, or roommate. It's not shocking news to know that *not communicating* with one another at dinner and watching TV instead while eating has affected relationship building in families.[7] In addition, *chewing food more slowly and putting your fork and knife down between bites spreads out the intake time so your brain has a chance to recognize the stomach is full.* You eat less this way. This was hard for me as well. I love eating fast, but now I make myself chew a few extra times and try to put my utensils down between bites to slow down! The result of eating without watching TV, for example, creates a positive association between eating well and feeling well. This is a stimulus that motivates you to continue healthful behavior because the result improves the **Feeling of Fullness.**

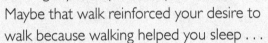

Positive Association

Do you remember a time
when you took a walk and
that night you slept soundly?
Maybe that walk reinforced your desire to
walk because walking helped you sleep . . .

How do you implement the changes? Well . . .
you build your own TOOLBOX!

You get to take charge and use tools, including cognitive behavior concepts using self-monitoring and improving self-efficacy by empowering yourself. We talked about goal setting, group support, behavioral substitution, stimulus control, energy intake (what you eat, physical activity and now—what so many don't recognize as important—restful sleep! You now have a wonderful opportunity to re-learn how to think about nutrition by changing your thoughts about food to better serve you. It's time to educate yourself on nutrition while keeping track of how you feel and inspiring self-awareness.

Survival Instinct Can Help You

You have survival instincts! The Cognitive Theory assumes that you value avoiding illness and that you expect that a specific behavior or activity will help you avoid a health problem or illness. You and I . . . all of us, make choices because we believe those choices will make a difference! This belief can motivate positive health behavior. Believing you are capable makes it possible for you to enjoy the journey and the process! Understand your body: there is no mechanism in your body that protects itself *against* over-eating, so it's your job to retrain it through new habits and positive rewards. The body does protect itself against starvation as it signals us to keep eating when we are starving, but unfortunately, *it does NOT tell us to STOP eating sugar, fats and treats even when we are overfed and storing all that food/sugar energy as FAT. Don't blame yourself,* go with it and try new ways of doing things to help your appetite and retrain the tummy-brain connection (more on this in upcoming chapters).

Other Surprises of food and social cues with SOCIALIZING!

I love socializing! And socializing makes me want to eat, because socializing and eating with family and friends have always been an amazingly wonderful positive experience. Every-time I see certain people/friends I crave a big plate of cheese, a glass of wine and cake! This happens even after having eaten dinner before I see them! Why? Conditioning! During many visits, we chatted over goat cheese, brie and a delectable bottle of Pinot. Yum. However, a few years ago I was more physically active and my metabolism was "peppier", so I burned it all up. Now it takes more work to stay in shape, so I have had to consciously *change my reactions to these "see friends eat a pound of cheese" cues.* I can still indulge with my friends, but stimulus controls have made me aware of my habits. Now, I am conscious of these external stimuli and eat only a small portion of goat cheese, a small glass of wine and a bite of cake, instead of the whole cheese wheel, well . . . most of the time! I may even skip the cake by not bringing dessert. By altering my behavior, I still indulge in the enjoyment and keep my waistline in check—even if at this stage of life, I have more curves! You may like to snack while talking to friends, like I do. For my favorite eat and chat sessions, I add chopped veggies to the cheese slices and no sugar, or high fiber crackers so that I eat more veggies than cheese and I still enjoy my cheese, but keep my mouth busy on the crunchy peppers and cooling cucumbers. There is always a fun new way to add and substitute while having a good time.

CHAPTER 2

Feeling Full

ENERGY INTAKE: CALORIES AND FEELING SATISFIED

Balance Based On You

AN AGE-OLD AND unfortunate focus with weight loss is the obsession on total *calories* and not calorie *quality* and *portion size*, both of which are contributors to feeling satisfied. Most of us gain weight when we eat more than our bodies burn, or when we eat foods that turn to sugar quickly (which makes us store belly fat) when they are more than we can utilize. However, *excessive focus on calories has not been useful or helpful when it comes to long-term health success.*

Who wants to keep counting calories day in and day out for 20 years—or even one year? Yes, I mentioned self-monitoring previously and the beneficial effects of initially counting calories. This is done to increase *awareness* so that you are *aware* of something

> Remember, no counting calories or weighing yourself if you have an eating disorder as these may contribute to unhealthier thought processes for you.

you might not realize regarding your calorie quantity, eating and weight. After this initial short-term exercise of counting calories (optional), you can move on to other self-monitoring activities.

Quality of Calories

Now, back to the quality of the calories. Imagine a potted plant without a drainage hole on the bottom of the pot. . . . If you keep pouring water into the pot, the dirt does not have a chance to dry out and can begin to mold and rot the roots. Well, *the same things happen to your body; you begin a decomposition process by overfeeding.* Your body experiences inflammatory reactions from excess calories, fats and sugars which you are not able to metabolize properly and end up stored as fat pockets:

Unused energy in the body, whether the source is protein, carbs, or fat, has to get stored and after muscles store all the extra glucose as glycogen (muscle fuel source), the rest gets stored as fat.

This seems logical. It is not just the calories that contribute to obesity, but the *excess* intake of calories that is the issue; so don't eliminate calories, as you need enough for energy. **Caloric needs change daily and depend on your activity level, genetics, stress levels, sleep quality and quantity and on your resting metabolic rate** (RMR—which is how many calories you burn while at rest).

In the next chapter will get into Intermittent Fasting. If you don't consume enough calories for your basic metabolic functions, you will slow down your basal metabolic rate in response to your body's attempt to conserving energy.

If you do not take in enough energy, your resting metabolic rate, responsible for up to 70% of your total energy expenditure (the calories you burn and need to function) drastically reduces by as much as 20%. In other words, if you don't

> BEWARE of not eating enough for long periods of time!
>
> Enough calories but Try Some Intermittent Fasting
>
> Intermittent Fasting can work to burn stored FAT and improve GLUCOSE levels!

eat enough, your body protects you and slows everything down to conserve energy. This results in rapidly *increasing* weight when you eat again, if you eat poor quality, high sugar, high saturated fat and low fiber foods. That is why unsustainable low-calorie diets don't work in the long run for most people, unless quality and quantity of food are tackled. The point is to eat when you are hungry, stop eating when you are satisfied (slow down, chew, pay attention, add fiber and feel full) and eat again when you are hungry (let your stomach tell you, not your emotions). There are also physiological factors to address when it comes to learning how to tell when you are full.

It's important to really understand that everyone's physiology is different

Avoid judging others based on their eating habits

There's nothing more annoying than a 'know-it-all'!

There is a tendency to "*need* to prove a point" or begin to lecture others once something has worked for us. Remember, what works for you isn't necessarily what works for someone else. Let others find their own paths.

Discover your own emotional eating cues and navigate your daily nutrition successfully.

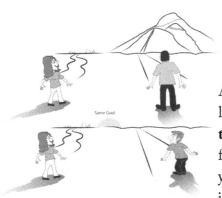

What's happening in your mind and belly?

As you make changes you learn how to **retrain your taste buds**, figure out your fullness cues and strengthen your digestion: Your Journey is *Your Journey.*

Each of us is a unique individual with a different chemical composition. That's why you must listen to your body!

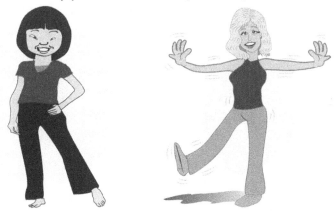

Personal Variations for Feeling Hungry

Some possibilities for feeling hungry after eating are: Glucose metabolism issues, acid reflux, poor insulin sensitivity (your insulin does not work well, your cells might not let glucose from your blood into your cells), poor digestion, other hormone and enzyme issues, hormone dysregulation, leptin (hormone to feel full), ghrelin (hormone to feel hunger), psychological triggers, imbalanced gut bacteria (microbiome), acid reflux and brain (feel good neurotransmitter) issues with serotonin (5-HT hydroxytryptamine receptors), or catecholamine may not be working optimally for you.[8]

Appetite Regulation and Fat Storage: LEPTIN and GHRELIN

Leptin is a hormone released by fat cells which helps decrease hunger in most of us. So that would mean, if leptin levels were higher, then we would feel fuller, or less hungry. However, those who suffer from obesity do not respond to their higher leptin levels and they still feel hungry. Though their leptin levels are often higher, their sensitivity to it is less and it *does not inhibit*

Get the Facts

Each of us is a unique individual with a different chemical composition.

Metabolism, fat usage and storage, and other biochemical factors related to metabolizing food and nutrients are complex.

In fact, there are over 400 known genes that affect overweight and obesity, including the FTO (obesity) genes and more.

That's why there is a whole study on Nutrigenomics (a whole other subject).

Here is a brief definition to satisfy your curiosity: *Nutrigenomics is the science and study of how specific genes increase the risk of chronic diseases, obesity, heart disease, cancers, strokes, and how foods interact with these genes' expressions.* . . .

A whole other book.

their hunger like it does in leaner individuals. On the bright side, a potential work around is to build up your own microbiome, and add probiotics. Probiotics have been shown to help regulate leptin sensitivity and obesity.[9] You can also add some grapefruit and rolled organic no added sugar oats to help with leptin sensitivity issues and add some bulk to your stomach (so you feel less hungry). Make your own **Probiotics** by eating foods considered to be **Prebiotics** (high fiber such as asparagus, or cabbage).

What about *Ghrelin? Ghrelin* affects hunger by telling you "You are hungry." It has a funny name, but the name comes from its role as a hormone: growth hormone-releasing peptide! If you

take a few letters from each word you get "**Ghrelin**". It is produced by the *ghrelinergic cells* in your stomach and pancreas and it
regulates appetite, but also is tasked to help the brain learn new
processes and adapt to changing external stimuli/environments.
I tell my students at the University to remember what ghrelin
does by thinking of their stomachs growling when they're hungry—the sound of growling and ghrelin can help you remember!
Hunger Fairy alert!

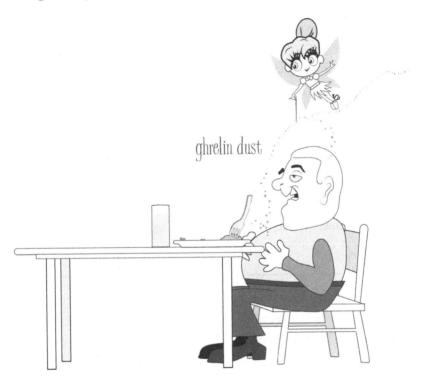

ghrelin dust

It seems that you can *learn* more when your stomach is empty, as
ghrelin is higher during non-eating times. Though it has found
its "fame" related to weight and appetite stimulation, ghrelin has
many more functions which affect not only fetal lung develop-
ment but is associated with decreased depression/anxiety and a
reduction in the production of insulin. As with all hormones, it

has many functions! For our purposes, keeping the Leptin and Ghrelin balance is important: When there are too many fat cells, havoc begins. We do our best to deal with the hunger that is experienced. How? Avoiding sugar spikes and appetite stimulation from too much sugar and not enough good fats, protein and plant based low sugar foods (not sugar free diet stuff).

What works? Decreasing foods that promote high insulin production such as sugars, refined flour and an inadequate intake of "make me full" foods such as protein, high fiber vegetables, high fiber grains (rolled oats or sprouted grain) and good oils (avocado, olives, olive oil, some saturated fats from coconut or real aged cheeses). Not everyone tolerates whole grains, so make sure you pay attention to how you feel after you eat whole grains (if you feel fatigued, bloated, tired, or hungrier, stick to more vegetables and proteins, choose low lectin foods as well, to protect your gut, intestinal lining and to control inflammation, hunger and weight).

Keeping your blood sugar steady (diabetic or not) helps reduce cravings, helps your brain work better and keeps you fuller longer by avoiding blood sugar highs and lows. Remember, your brain is 60% fat: it likes the good stuff, it's okay to have healthy fats (olive oil, avocado, walnuts) https://www.ncbi.nlm.nih.gov/pmc/articles/PMC6603809/ .

Feeling Full with Fiber

If you cannot feel full, you can add two tablespoons of oat bran to eight to twelve ounces of water and follow it with another glass of water: the fiber expands in the stomach.[10] If you have Celiac Disease, use a non-grain fiber such as flax meal. This helps with that strange empty gnawing sensation in the stomach. Like my patients, I have found that certain foods trigger my hunger. Sugar and potatoes are major hunger triggers for me. If I have them in my meal, I often notice a quick hunger crash following my meal even after having had a ton of protein and fiber and salad; the glucose and insulin reactions in my body make these foods a hunger-trigger for me. This understanding is a part of my journey and my self-discovery towards managing my own appetite and hunger. A fix for me: I use ½ cup of cooked brown Basmati or white Basmati rice instead of potatoes, skip the sugar and double the green vegetable.

You will have your own road map and your own fix it tips related to what works and what does not work for you. Watch for the signs and chart your course.

To satiate hunger, some of my patients do what I do with the water and oat bran before each meal in order to feel fuller physically *before* they eat. You can also do this before eating. Stomach acid levels or biochemical gastro-intestinal cues send the brain a sense of satiation from the expanding fiber in your gut and a feeling of satisfaction. **NOT** all fiber does this and you still need to eat regular food not just fiber. These fibers have been shown to help with satiety: **β-glucan,** lupin kernel fiber, rye bran, whole grain rye, or a mixed high-fiber.[11]

A study on fasting reported by Jarrar and The National Institutes of Health confirmed that 11g fiber per ~90 grams of product of Soho helped decrease hunger, satiety and improved lipid profiles during fasting periods.

How do you find out what foods may be affecting you? Try keeping a journal for 30 days to track daily hunger responses. Sometimes, it is not a psychological battle of mind over matter, but rather, a *physiological* factor that plays a role in your eating habits. A multitude of factors affect weight, so please don't judge yourself by others. Learn from yourself and others: Be wise. You get to make the choices!

Get the Facts

Fullness Tips[55]

- Add fiber to six to eight ounces of water before eating if you are struggling. Try

- **β-glucan**, lupin kernel fiber, rye bran, whole grain rye, or mixed high-fiber.

- Add fiber-rich foods, especially vegetables to each meal to help with satiety.

- Avoid foods that turn to sugar quickly and may make you dump insulin into your system, which in turn may lower your blood sugar too quickly. People who have diabetic parents or family members are at greater risk of developing diabetes. Pay more attention to these potential hunger triggers, as not everyone reacts the same to sugar, corn syrup, or high carbohydrate meals. Remember, it is your own biochemical reaction, and you should be honest with yourself about how you feel physically.

- Try lean protein, high fiber, and plant fat (avocado) for breakfast and test your appetite two and three hours post breakfast, lunch, or dinner. Some people do well with ½ cup cooked rolled oats—but that is not true for everyone. Add nuts to this to keep you full longer as they digest more slowly, are a great protein, have fiber, and provide good fats, but they do not spike your blood glucose, which is a good thing.

- Keep a food log to determine how quickly you get hungry after eating. If it is quick, then you may need a new type of food. Some people get hungry after pancakes, but not after scrambled eggs. Eggs are protein, digest more slowly, and may keep you full longer without a glucose spike.

- Try Intermittent Fasting (eat dinner and lunch—skip breakfast—or eat breakfast and late lunch, skip dinner: Not eating for 16 to 18 hours, but eating regular meals within the six to eight hours left over) helps avoids hunger in the long run. You are allowing your body to NOT overproduce insulin. Since during fasting there is not a high level of glucose in your blood for which insulin is required, you may experience (after adjusting to this of course), incredible appetite control. If you are diabetic, on Medications, or Injecting Insulin, you must speak with your physician about the fasting schedule, and you may NOT be a candidate for it. ALWAYS take your health condition into account.

- Practice paying attention to chewing, the taste of your food, and taking that time to sit quietly and eat your meal, instead of multi-tasking and gulping, as that technique does not allow for appropriate digestions and gut-mind satiety recognition. You may not even notice you have eaten if you are doing something else. This attention is a form of mindfulness.

- Avoid eating in front of the TV as you will eat 30%-150% more than you might have eaten otherwise.

- Avoid packaged foods as they contain more fillers, gums, and appetite triggers. Try fresher, foods. If they are frouncesen vegetables, or frouncesen protein without fillers, and sauces you will have less risk of adding appetite triggers purposely put in there so you would eat more. This is just part of food science and production, but you want to advocate for yourself.

- Replace high sugar drinks with healthy alternatives—water and lemon vs juice or soda— this will save you six to twelve teaspoons of sugar, added calories, and a potential increase in your blood glucose sugar. Have an orange instead of the juice as a glass of juice is made with about four to eight oranges.

- Studies on nine 14-year-old children reported that fruit drinks resulted in increased food intake. (https://www.mdpi.com/2072-6643/11/2/270)

- Have fun Enjoy and Laugh!

CHAPTER 3

Exercise Miracles

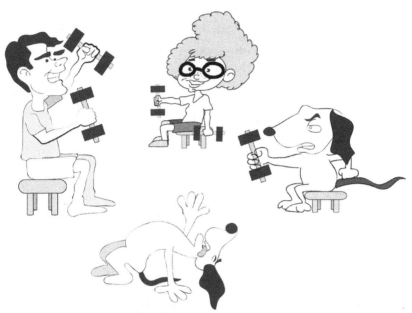

Physical Activity

WE HAVE ALL heard this: walk and exercise . . . bla, bla, bla. Yup, it's true and as much as we can be nagged about it, we certainly can't change the reality of physiology and exercise. Remember when you felt great after a hike, even if something might have been a bit achy? How about that awesome high after a tennis match, or a bike ride, or the memory of playing in the park as a kid? If we can tap into the good vibes of being active, then the thought of exercise will not be a punishment, but instead, a wonderful expression and reminder of youthful memories and feeling great. On that note, let's talk about why the proverbial "do your exercise" meme really works.

Exercise and an active lifestyle *do* expend energy by burning calories, suppressing appetite, preventing and managing hypertension, reducing the risk of obesity, diabetes, serum cholesterol, abdominal fat storage and other cardiovascular health issues. *WOW*, now, that's a good list. We know that any physical activity and exercise have a multitude of benefits and here they are: improved psychological health, lean body mass (muscle), enhanced metabolism and a cyclical reinforcement that helps you continue a healthy lifestyle. Did you know that exercise is associated with a reduction in cancer risk as well as a deterrent against depression and lethargy—that feeling of "Oh my gosh, I am not moving, or getting off this couch?"

SO, WHY DON'T WE DO IT!

Well, we know the list of barriers, don't we? It includes time, money, living in unsafe locations, too tired, too much work, busy with the kids, feeling uncomfortable, self-consciousness and the list goes on—and to add to these annoying emotional and environmental barriers, in 2020, the shutting down of gyms due to SARS-CoV2 virus put another nail on that coffin! So, what seems to help us get started?

FIND A BUDDY

One pound of body fat = 3,500 calories. BUT that doesn't mean you will lose weight just by burning 3,500 cal.

Types of calories do different things to fat storage! Try some intermittent fasting—at least 12 hours of not eating: One example is to fast between 8 p.m. to 8 a.m. Drink plenty of water, ask your doctor if you are able to do this, monitor how you feel, keep a journal and try a few hours at a time. More on this in your next chapter!

When not doing intermittent fasting . . . eat enough to support your metabolism and lean body mass—keep your muscles fed.

Generally speaking, we do not want you to go below 1,200 calories per day (unless your physician is monitoring you and has prescribe this, or on occasional 500 calorie intermittent fasting days) as this may slow down your metabolism as a protective mechanism done to keep you alive.

Once a Calorie, always a Calorie: Don't hate the calorie!

CALORIES: You need a range from 20 to 30 calories per kilogram (kilograms) of energy per day. To get kilograms, divide your weight in pounds by 2.2. Generally, 1,200 calories are the basic metabolic needs per day for a woman of average height and size (your needed fuel to function) and for men it is 1,800 calories. The reduction in calories can come from consuming less and increasing calories burned through exercise. You need calories to survive and as always, moderation and self-awareness are vital keys.

Any exercise is better than no exercise!

EXERCISE: The basic recommendation is 5 hours of moderate to vigorous exercise per week and according to the American Heart Association, at least 150 minutes of moderate cardio, or 75 minutes of intense cardio (runners). You can check out their website here https://www.heart.org/en/healthy-living/fitness/fitness-basics/aha-recs-for-physical-activity-infographic. Twenty minutes of interval exercise (interval exercise is changing the pace from slow to fast to slow and back) three times per week makes a difference, as long as you use intermittent high-speed 30-second bursts to engage all

> **Fun Fact**
>
> "Skinny" people who do not exercise have greater risk of cardiovascular death, than overweight people who exercise regularly! See, exercise is your friend, and a stroll around some green trees supports your mental health as well—two for one.

your muscle fibers (slow twitch, fast twitch, superfast twitch). Regular exercise helps decrease sudden death from cardiovascular disease, no matter what weight you are! [12]

If you live in a concrete jungle, get outside for some fresh air and watch YouTube Green Walk, or Ocean Beach walk images and video streaming, as this will also get your brain in that safer, healthier space. Here is a link I found of the Flying Dutchman YouTube channel that has a VIRTUAL tree walk and it is titled, *"Redwood The Boy Scout Tree Trail 4K Walk (*https://www.youtube.com/watch?v=o-xoBW9NZNI).

Note: I am not sponsored by or being paid by this YouTube channel, I simply wrote down in the YouTube search bar "tree hike" and this one appeared. It's perfect!

Now, what about our muscles? I know mine are not as pumped up as I wished they were and as I have gotten older, the length of time my muscles stay toned is *getting shorter and shorter* (hormone levels change), so I need to keep working on that muscle group. I also need to remember that I have slow, fast and superfast twitch muscles that need to be engaged for a more rounded approach to fitness. Now, would I rather binge on my favorite Netflix show? Oh, yes! But . . . I also love feeling fit and I know I will end up feeling way more energized if I give myself at least 30 minutes of dance or a fast walk—which ends up helping me eat less and feel friendlier—less grumpy.: That's always a plus at work and around your mates, or spouse. That *'whole mind and benefits game'* works; gentle reminders are tasty treats for the soul, then I can watch Netflix.

Want to burn fat? Use all your muscle fibers!

**USE ALL MUSCLE FIBER TYPES
to SHAPE YOUR BODY**

Slow/Fast/Super-fast

YOU only use fast and superfast muscle types when you do sprints and quick bursts of exercise for 30 seconds—these are the movements that help you burn more fat! Walking trains and works out your "slow twitch" muscle fibers. Your heart also needs for you to train its fast twitch muscle fibers for ultimate heart health! You can walk, dance, garden, hike, or ride a bike . . . *and* . . . you *should implement intermittent speeds* when you do these activities to fire all muscle-twitch fibers! To create a daily activity level—you've heard this one before, "park far away from the entrance to a building, take the stairs," and walk around the block at different speeds before or after work or even on your lunch break, or march around in your living room while watching your favorite TV show! Be sure to change the speed of what you do to engage all three muscle twitch fibers! Every bit of energy expenditure helps you burn calories to stay in good shape. Don't trap yourself into thinking " . . . if you don't train like an Olympic athlete, then it's not worth trying at all." Not much fat will be burned if you do not get your heart rate up to about 70% of your *target heart rate* (hint: 220 minus your age = Number, multiply that by 70% to 75%. This is the best way to start burning some fat through target heart rate cardio exercise!) For example, if you are 50 years old you follow this formula to calculate your heart rate: 220 - 50 = 170 x 70% (.070) = 119. The basic formula is 220 - (your age), times the percent heart rate you want to calculate (ACE Fit | Heart Rate Zone Calculator acefitness.org/).

CDC and BUMMER STATS on US cardio fitness

Unfortunately, the CDC (Centers for Disease Control)[13] reports a consistent decrease in total physical activity in Americans and speculates it is related to increased work hours, increased television viewing, computers and a reduction in available physical activity for children in schools. Not kidding, right?! Even though more people belong to gyms now than ever, the total energy output is not meeting the excess total energy (calories) input, nor is it training the body and heart. Remember that funny photo of people taking the escalator on the way to their gym's entrance? If you are going to the gym, might as well take those ten steps! So funny. Those stairs engage some of your twitch muscles as they contract and will help you build a bit of muscle mass—maybe not as activated through a flat treadmill. If you are physically able, go ahead, take the stairs! Avoid the escalator and take that flight of stairs in front of your gym!

Another unfortunate denial strategy we use is that a few minutes of exercise can handle all the extra sugar drinks we consume. On that note, take a look at the following table.

Fun Fact: Exercise and Calories

Based on Activity at 3.5 miles per hour

Food	Calories	Time to Burn
1 can of soda: 12 ounces	111	25-minute fast walk
1 cup vanilla ice cream	280	60-minute fast walk
2 tablespoons Honey	120	30-minute fast walk
1 orange juice: 8 ounces	100	22-minute fast walk

It's true, we are encouraged to take walks during our lunch break. However, what if those walks are so slow, our heart rate barely goes up? Well, in that case, the benefit is not burning fat, but rather improving basic circulation and getting out of the office. Both, which are good. On the other hand, you really want to increase your heart rate if you want to train the heart, as well as build muscle mass and burn fat. Get that heart rate up; monitor your pulse (fit bit or phone app for android and iPhones). Do your calculation: 220 minus your age, times 70%, then you know what your pulse should be so you can have that "training burning fat walk."

Next time you walk on a treadmill, gradually increase the speed up to 3.5 mph (carefully and work up to it from 2.0 mph) and notice that increasing heart rate. Then put it back to 2.0 mph and notice the difference. As you adapt to increasing your speed to help reach your target heart rate, you will reap the weight loss, hip strengthening and mood lifting benefits. The more trained and fit you are, the higher the intensity or speed, but be sure to monitor your joint pain, and do only what you tolerate. Some people are fine at 5.0 mph, and others are better off and trained well at 3.5 mph. Listen to your body.

Let's talk about those extra sugary drinks. If you have 32 ounces of a juice or soda, how many calories might that be? Here is your answer: 400 calories or more. That means you have to walk at 3.5 mph for 22 minutes FOUR times that day to keep those calories and sugar from potentially being stored as fat in your adipose (fat) cells. That's 88 minutes! **Important**: You do not automatically gain weight from adding 400 calories, but you will gain weight and stored fat if these 400 calories are part of *over consumption (above your needs)*, as anything in excess, over time, will be converted to fat for storage. Again, *Balance*.

Don't obsess about calories! Focus on the Moderation and Quality of your Food!

EXERCISE ANOREXIA and OBSESSION

Don't get into the danger zone of eating and over-exercising whereby every calorie is counted and every minute of exercise is calculated to burn those calories—that is a type of eating and over-exercising disorder—even without counting calories. We call this anorexia athletica or hypergymnasia (sports anorexia).

DANGER ZONE AND MORE OBSESSION

Obsession with types of foods and fear of what they will do to your body is termed orthorexia. But, if you are not at risk of eating disorders and do not have a history of eating disorder, you can pay attention to calories at first, but then LET IT GO, once you have learned a little bit about food and your body. This is geared more for overweight and obese individuals who may have diabetes or chronic health conditions who have never really paid attention to food and its composition and how these may affect their body. On that note, did you know you can burn 300 calories on a moderate-paced 1 ½ hour hike? During this hike, you will not only be burning calories, but you will also be building muscle, strengthening your bones and relieving stress by being physically active, with the added bonus of being in NATURE. Calories burned (per time-period) are an average calculation. Every person, depending on their physiology, size, age, muscle mass and gender will burn calories and stored fat at different rates, so do not depend on the "calories burned on the exercise machine." Your body will let you know what's working and what isn't. Again, once you have a basic understanding, **STOP COUNTING** calories and fat and relax on the over exercising.

Enjoy life, like your body, accept changes,

but be honest about your health and well-being.

Muscles and Human Growth Hormones

From the time I started writing this book, to a couple of years later when my body started changing in this amazingly life-altering middle age time period, I have had to put to practice the advice I am giving you. It is no longer coming from observing patient or knowledge of books or studies, but from personal experiences of a changing human body, with its hormone changes, physical changes and energy changes. Oh my goodness! What a great blessing to be able to be REAL about this information. I am not using a ghost writer and I am not using other researchers to do the work for me. What I present to you are from my real-life experiences, my 20 plus years of seeing nutrition patients and my active peer reviewed academic *gobbledygook* painstaking hours of research. I have neither been spoon-fed results or data, nor have I delegated the work to someone else. Editing and proofreading, of course, is a must and done by other helpful God-sent angels. Here we go on Human Growth Hormone.

As we age, we produce less human growth hormone (HGH), less testosterone, progesterone and estrogen which all affect lean body mass and fat storage. As we get older, we need to purposely create and build more lean muscle. More lean muscle helps us burn more calories throughout the day. A regular regime of muscle-strengthening and building will not only help reduce our excess fat storage but will also help strengthen our bones and decrease our risk of osteoporosis as an added useful bonus!

Just 3 times per week, 20 minutes each time, can help improve muscle mass and protect your bone density. Resistance training and a few jumps here and there, adequate **Vitamin D** intake (sun, supplements, foods) are all protective against bone loss—even as we lose weight, or as we get older. Check out this link by NIH: https://www.ncbi.nlm.nih.gov/pmc/articles/PMC4217506/. Keep up to date on your terms as well.

My Message to You
Eat Well, and Be Merry, Dance, and Drink Water, and Laugh!

There is no doubt that eating more veggies improves our health, and there is no doubt that excess meat and processed food can contribute to health issues, just like excess soda and sugar drinks increase weight and inflammatory processes. This is why I encourage all of you to take charge of your health, make changes that make you feel great, and listen to your body. Always try new things, and don't punish yourself—laughter, play, and good food are a great balance. Enjoy your health.

CHAPTER 4

Sleep, Stress, Lights and Weight Loss

Sleep, Stress and Weight Loss
Sleep Some Weight Off

MY PATIENTS ARE always surprised to learn that sleep or lack of sleep affects weight. For example, studies on sleep and its effect on weight or BMI (Body Mass Index) remind us that each aspect benefits from the other. In one study 98 participants were followed for three months with a follow-up assessment after ten months.[14] It turned out that sleep duration, body composition (shape/fat storage), what you ate during the day, exercise and weight *were all associated with each other* and *getting enough sleep was essential for weight management*. Not sleeping enough could make you eat more and eating more could make you sleep less. Sleeping helped you burn fat. However, sleeping excessively (more than 12 hours) could slow you down and contribute to weight gain! So, what does this all mean: **You** get to pay attention to your energy, your body and how sleep is affecting your mood, appetite and energy. It all matters. If you are not sleeping enough, work on some tricks through guided mediation, sound therapy and putting your phone in another room, avoiding stressful people if you can and being aware of what **DOES HELP** you get the rest you need.

So, what else do these sleep studies tell us? Here is what they found:
Those who followed a healthy diet and slept about
9 hours per night averaged 10% weight loss.

I know, the last time I slept nine hours was . . . I can't even remember the decade!

Let's continue with the cool data: Participants who slept fewer than 7 hours, as you might expect, experienced less weight loss. In addition, lack of sleep is associated with more stress, which often leads to high blood pressure and poor health choices. Okay, no surprise there. Since our bodies are complex, mysterious and filled with wonderful chemicals that are interrelated, it is important to understand that among multiple chemicals and enzymes, at least these two appetite controlling hormones, **leptin** and **ghrelin**, are disrupted by too little sleep.

**Those who sleep less also have an increased
risk in heightened appetite and obesity.**[15]

The balance of activities, food intake, when and what you eat, hours of rest and exercise as well as the people that surround you contribute to your overall wellness.

You are a complete being: Your body is not separate from your mind, nor is your spiritual wellness separate from your body or mind.

INTERNET AND SOCIAL MEDIA ADDICTION

Electronics Addiction Sleep Disruption!

For the majority of surveyed and studied people, things that disrupt sleep include caffeine, stress, lack of exercise, TV and all electronic equipment, including phones used to check email, text, Facebook (FB) and social media used continually throughout the day. The light impulses, brain activity and physiological responses created by our electronic dependence have been shown to keep some people awake longer, reducing restful and total sleep. Brain scan evidence has contributed to this fascinating reality which is true for many people. If you are a video gamer, it is critical to know that a study showed on-line video game players who played video games before sleep had reduced REM (rapid eye movement) sleep and had a harder time going to sleep (faster heart rates and brain activity).[16] REM sleep is important for the deepest rest, where we also do a lot of cellular repair. Here is another cool one.: A study of 532 adults found that insomnia and daytime sleepiness was associated with using the computer, watching TV, video games, mobile phones and audio players.[17]

It's true! I had to stop using HULU, Netflix and Amazon Prime at 11 p.m. and had to start working on my late night "I want to chill with the BBC and watch my "Poirot and Miss Marple who-dunits" addiction. I must admit, I do sleep more hours if I turn the TV and iPad off and instead read a few paragraphs of a book. Reading certainly helps you relax and go to sleep. Give it a try and see how it goes. It does work for me and has worked for many of my 30-year-olds, as well as my very stressed hard working full-time job mothers in their 40s and 50s.

**The extra sleep will help you reach your
health goals more readily.**

Discipline is not just exercise, but also self-care so you can function!

Managing time is important, if you know you have to get up at 6 a.m. and you are also in school, like I had been during the Ph.D. program, **advice given to me** was to avoid time lost through social media and TV if you notice it is affecting your sleep. One behavioral therapist with whom I worked told me to set a timer when I start with FB or anything else and stop when the timer goes off, instead of wasting hours of the day, or valuable minutes that could be used for something healthy and productive. There is online FB social media promotion, Instagram™, Twitter™ , Snapchat™ and more, but it is important to give that a rest as well, just like leaving work at 5 or 6 p.m., there needs to be a stopping point of self-promotion, anger and sad stories! Even 5 hours of cat videos need a break!

ONLINE MENTAL HEALTH, SLEEP AND WEIGHT

YouTube, Facebook, Instagram, Twitter and More . . .

Computer and phone addiction can affect not only your sleep but your overall emotional health. A Swedish study looking at over 4,100 men and women over the course of a year found increased *mental health consequences* with mobile phone and texting use. What does "Mental Health Consequences" mean? The results showed increased anxiety, increased depression and reduced sleep with increased use of phones and texting; the more mobile phone and texting occurred the greater the negative effects.[18] Our new FOMO—fear of missing out word—has gotten its claim to fame for so many reasons. Here is another FOMO research result: An article in the Daily Mail of the United Kingdom reported increased social media use reduced time for physical activity, increased guilt and stress over not looking at FB or other online messaging and increased stress and anxiety overall.[19] Online activities included messaging, checking personal messages, gaming and any social-media activity, even for work related access, effect quality of sleep and well-being.

Those who were expected to be available 24 hours a day by mobile phone had higher stress and anxiety than those not required to be available. I know, obvious, but hey, unless it's studied, "it's not real." Right?!

The average number of minutes on social media a day is just 2 hours and 22 minutes.) (https://review42.com/social-media -marketing-statistics/) Can you imagine how much exercise or outdoor activities you could do if you were actually moving— even if you split the difference—you could still get 1 hour of exercise in a day.

What do you think the average time spent logged in to FB is in the U.S.? Wrenn reported that users spent an average of 75 min- utes on FB, logged in at least six times per day, logged in every time they started their computer and that 26% of the people

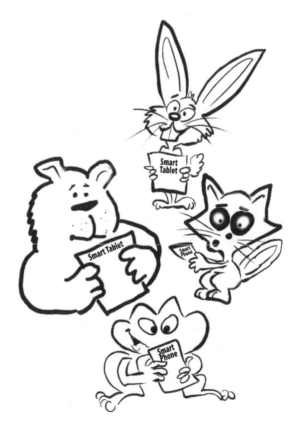

felt "ill at ease" if they did not check their computer (stress from pressure to reply, or stress from missing something).[20] That was a few years ago. What about in 2020? Recent data tells us there an additional split of time between FB (https://sproutsocial.com /insights/facebook-stats-for-marketers/) and Instagram https:// www.brandwatch.com/blog/youtube-stats/ (owned by FB), with 74% of FBers checking in daily and watching eight billion videos per day. In Canada FB is the most popular platform used at 83%, with 18- to 24-year-olds using all social media the most. (https:// papers.ssrn.com/sol3/papers.cfm?abstract_id=3651206#:~:text= %2D%20Facebook%20remains%20the%20most%20popular ,%25)%20and%20Instagram) Canadians, according to 2020 Statistica analysis, spent at least 2 hours per day between social media and use of game consoles, offsetting potential for exercise. This does not include their reported additional 3.2 hours per day of video streaming, television etc. What might the health risks be?

It may seem harmless, but is it? As of October 2020, eye opening data from Omnicore, reveal YouTube™ viewing statistics with a whopping 2 billion monthly active users, 30 million daily active users, a minimum of 40 minutes a day of viewing per person and over a billion videos watched per day. Once you put movies, streaming, YouTube, FB, Twitter, Instagram etc. together, you can imagine how little time might be left for exercise, especially after school or work. (https://www.omnicoreagency.com /youtube-statistics/) and (https://www.brandwatch.com/blog /youtube-stats/)

COMPUTERS AND YOUR WEIGHT: COMPUTER TUMMY ALERT!

Sleep duration does affect weight and your sleep is affected by use of your stuff! Electronics/technology such as TV, mobile phones, video games and internet use can "mess you up!"[21] Here is an example of 632 susceptible adolescents studied in the UK.; The longer or more frequent the technology use (mobile phone, tablets etc.), the less sleep they had and the higher their weight and BMI was. Those who used technologies less, had improved sleep and were generally normal weight and sometimes underweight.[22] It's like watching too much TV or doing too much on your bottom—a dilemma for editors and sound engineers, mixers and the whole digital entertainment industry. My YouTube videos take my lovely editor hours to do! What do you do then? Be aware and **add** the time to do cardio and build muscle, otherwise you will unfortunately suffer the consequences of a weaker CORE—increased risk of low back and disc issues, weight gain, obesity, diabetes, cardiovascular disease, depression, anxiety and the list goes on. Of course, not every single person will react this way, but statistically speaking, the **TREND** is undeniable and shows an **UPWARD TREND** of increased time on social media and computers and increased obesity risk.

Social Media Stress Party! How Do You Socialize Now?

The total stress overload and time used for social media and computer activities disrupt valuable time otherwise available for physically interacting with others. This includes speaking with others on the phone or in person vs. texting and not engaging, taking time to cook or exercise and experience the outdoors. Logically, the more you engage in mobile phone and computer activities, the less physical activity you are going to experience and the less likely you are to prepare something yummy in the kitchen.

It only takes 15 to 25 minutes to have a healthy fresh vegetable, fruit and protein, or nut and fruit snack or meal.

Try an Internet break, get up stretch your legs, take a deep breath and take a nice ten minutes to eat a fresh apple or a chopped salad with almonds, have a handful of walnuts and a spring time apricot.

Your Voluntary Love Assignment: Pay attention to how much time you are spending on the computer and mobile phones with respect to social media. Note how you feel about using the cell phone, need to respond immediately to chats or texts and how many times you check FB or other sites that may hijack your time. Observe the sites and their content and their effect on your mood, hunger, energy and anxiety levels. Most importantly, notice how it may be affecting your sleep time. Have a good self-analysis week!

> **NOTE:** It's not only sleep, but how all these things work together to influence how you interact with **other** people, especially when you get involved in negative and angry banter on social media. Take a breath . . . and take a mental health break. You might find the love again and even share a little laughter.

TRACKING SLEEP AND SOCIAL MEDIA SHEET

Sleep and Social Media Tracking

Make up your own Tracking Sheet that is useful to you.

List how you feel: angry, annoyed, pissed-off, resentful, happy, excited, etc., Number of times you logged into Social Media, gaming, chats, texts, etc., Time, in minutes, you spent in chats, texts, messaging, using email, and surfing the web. When listing your sleep time, track what time you went to sleep and what time you woke up. You can write anything you want that you want to notice in your personalized chart.

Day, Date and Day of the Week	I Feel Like*	Social Media Visits	Duration of any Electronic Check-ins	Rest

*Make note of any mood patterns you experience.

CHAPTER 5

Your Brain and Your Weight

MEET YOUR BRAIN

Trends, Food and Your Brain

You can make a difference in your health for life!

I OFTEN HEAR comments like, "We all have to die sometime, I might as well enjoy myself, so I'll do what I want now. It's too expensive to eat well. My family won't eat the good stuff! I don't

Happy Brain

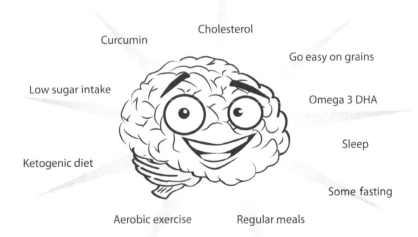

Cholesterol

Curcumin

Go easy on grains

Low sugar intake

Omega 3 DHA

Sleep

Ketogenic diet

Some fasting

Aerobic exercise   Regular meals

want to cook two meals. You don't understand, my life is too hard! There's no good food when I travel for work," and many other health sabotaging, fear-based though legitimate, overwhelmed thought responses. Over the years I have learned how to help clients *reframe* those thoughts. Hey, I have to work on my own thoughts too. Now, to address the "we've all 'gotta' die sometime" response. I want to emphasize the quality of life; not longevity with ill health but longevity with good health. For many of my pleasantly surprised clients, change can be less difficult, less expensive and less overwhelming than they imagined. For some, making a list of all the extra dollars spent on sodas, chips, alcohol, cigarettes, fancy/expensive coffees and even gambling, allowed them to reallocate those funds to healthier, more filling foods. This was money they *already had* but were not using *wisely*—to promote their health. It *does* take a leap of faith and at times, even a cheerleader. So why not surround yourself with cheerleaders?

For larger families on a budget, adding brown rice vs. white rice, carrots vs chips, black beans vs white bread can maintain a budget and add improved nutrients.

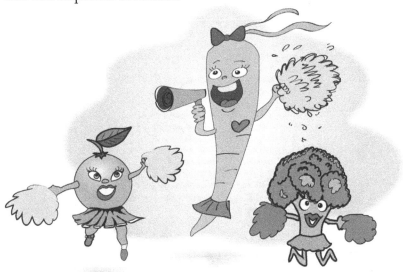

There is no doubt that having a support group with people around you who are positive and not critical and who believe in you will *make an incredible difference*. That also means that our behavior and attitudes also affect and influence *others* and we can also be their *cheerleaders*. Remember how it felt when someone criticized you? Not super motivational right? What about your words, do you pay attention to what you say or think about others and about yourself? It's something to think about.

HEALTH TRENDS THAT CONTRIBUTE TO DISEASE

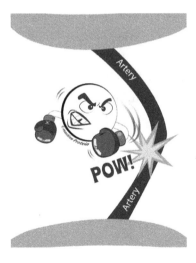

Oh no, more information—but this is *cool*. We want to feel great; I want to feel great; you want to feel great. Okay, so what do we know? What are these indicators of disease? Red flags of health issues include increased levels of triglycerides in your blood (literally too much fat in your blood). Stored fat around your liver results in high liver enzymes which means your liver is compromised. Increased C-reactive protein informs us you have inflammation. Disease causing inflammation is not good (period). This can lead to lazy, confused organs and even under the skin (our "favorite"— cellulite and fat rolls).

By the time we see our weight gain, it's not just the visible fat that makes us feel "yucky", but the excess fat in the secret chambers around our organs that contribute to the consequences and increase our health risks. *We* should strive for a healthy and active lifestyle because wellness makes all the difference in the quality of our lives. When we feel good, we have more energy to continue healthful choices and the more energy we have means we have the potential to fulfill our dreams! Even 5 minutes of marching in place between tasks can help.

What are your dreams and aspirations? Write them down and make them real in your mind—then see yourself making them happen. What is on your *Bucket List*? Do you want to learn a new language, go to dance classes, join a swim team, enroll in a painting class, go back to school, have a baby, volunteer, write short stories, learn to sing, or ride horses? Mine was jumping out of an airplane. I know, crazy, but facing my fear of heights and doing that tandem SkyDive Madrid jump (start at 2.47 minutes https://youtu.be/ogkFWcry-uo) was one of the coolest things I had ever done. For all of us, good health provides the foundation to gain the benefits of a clear mind and the energy to achieve our dreams and goals. It is a cyclical relationship: Maintain a healthy life to maintain a healthy weight for a happy, healthy life! Remember, we are not talking about skinniness, or extreme fitness, we are talking about Health and Wellbeing and we all know what that is—forget the extremes, enjoy the reality. That includes letting our brains function . . . and one of the most "fog up your brain" contributors is *excess sugar* . . .

Now, for *your brain and sugar* . . . .

Why should you care about high sugar intake?

Because sugar shuts off your brain!

Yes, your brain lives on glucose, but that does not mean you should drink gallons of it!

Small amounts of sugar intake can be metabolized by the body, but when you consume more sugar than your body uses through daily activity or that it can tolerate, then the body loses its balance

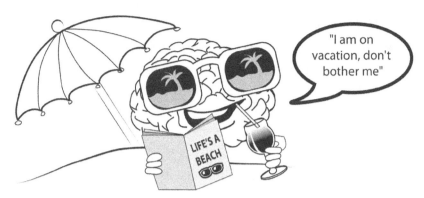

and a cascade of potentially unhealthful issues begin. You know the drill! Taking a vacation is great, but when your brain takes a vacation, that's another story. On that note, researchers have found that an important chemical function that your brain performs is *decreased* when you consume too much sugar. Your brain goes on vacation which is never a good thing!

When this *brain-derived neurotropic factor* (aka: BDNF) is low from too much sugar intake, guess what happens? There is an increased possibility of depression, dementia and an inability to *know when to stop eating*!!! Your whole "fullness" sensors *turn off!* You might be creating a viscous cycle of sugar cravings while decreasing feelings of fullness by chemically altering your physiology with high sugar intake. Sadly, you probably never suspect the sabotage.

MEET YOUR BRAIN! BE NICE TO EACH OTHER.

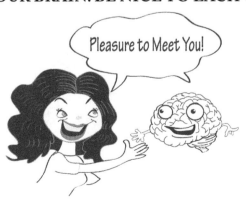

Oxytocin, Paxil, Sugar and Sex

How about that Oxytocin? We have all heard about drugs that increase the Oxytocin effect and that are used in treating depression and anxiety, such as the prescription Paxil. But the most fun way to increase Oxytocin is *sex*. Of course, if you have been married a long time and forgot to have sex, make sure you plan a little bit of fun with your spouse, as this sexy neurotransmitter will help you *bond* and feel the flutters of "I love you honey" again, and burn 70–100 calories, not a bad thing, right?![23] Your partner will love you for it. Now, here's the kicker:

Chronic sugar intake affects oxytocin regulation.

When it comes to *feeling full*, oxytocin helps you feel full. Normal levels of oxytocin keep you satisfied. Guess what happens when you allow your sweet tooth to indulge in daily high doses of sugar or high-fructose corn syrup? You end up reducing oxytocin cells and as a result, you don't feel satisfied, which means, you *don't feel full*. We know what it does for your *satiety*; if you eat loads of sugar over prolonged periods, you will most likely be messing up that brain pathway making it harder for you to feel full. High sugar intake seems to degrade the biochemical pathways that help you feel full and satisfied, not only through oxytocin levels but also through brain growth hormones.[24]

Oxytocin is a Superhero for You!
BIONIC BRAIN CELLS

Oxytocin regulates a myriad of stuff in your brain, including memories associated with your sense of smell: Your memory is triggered through smell. Smells trigger all kinds of food memories for me, as well as emotional reactions based on good, gross and wonderful things! What about this Brain Growth Hormone? Well, our brain cells need help too, just like our muscles and the rest of our cells and recently, I think I need *way more help* for my brain as the years accumulate . . . The growth hormone, **BDNF (Brain Derived Neurotrophic Factor)**, helps regenerate brain cells, aids memory and reduces cognitive deterioration. Again, I could use some increase please: more BDNF, thank you!

It's no surprise then, that when we look at brain chemistry, it is this infamous BDNF that's deficient in Alzheimer's and Parkinson's patients. We all need some brain regeneration! . . . and if you are old enough, you will remember the TV show, The *Six Million Dollar Man*— not so much with inflation now— maybe, we should rename the show the Billion Dollar Man, or Lindsey Wagner in the BIONIC woman. These fictional super humans had extra-human powers through android-like artificially enhanced human limbs. Our bodies are remarkable. They can *regenerate* cells and tissues—our livers, our brains—are our own lizard-like regenerators.

So, obviously having *more* BDNF is protective. But here's the kicker: *Not only does excess sugar reduce BDNF, excess food intake also reduces BDNF.* Again, we see the benefits of not overeating (hard to do with my Italian heritage, I love food). Of course, we see studies verifying that eating less seems to **INCREASE** this beautiful brain growth hormone![25] This is yet another reminder as to the potential brain benefits, amongst so many others, of occasional intermittent fasting. It appears that overeating and excess sugar intake not only affect weight and elevate the risk of diseases like diabetes, but they also affect brain function and chemistry. Like the body, the brain is dependent on food intake, but obviously, overfed bodies are not happy either. We know nutrition affects our health, but it was commonly assumed the brain would not be affected. Who knows why we were so myopic? For example, among many tidbits about food and our bodies, we now know that poor nutrition is also associated with aggravating

Attention Deficit Disorder.[26] IQ is influenced by essential fats in utero (mama eating good oils early improved IQ and concentration levels of babies later). So, remember, eating right is important for your brain as well as your body.

Your brain depends on what you eat, just like your car depends on the materials from which it is made, the gas which powers it and the lubricants which keep it running.

Eat a balanced diet with protein, good fats and slowly absorbed carbohydrates vs. high sugars and fast food and you will feel better (because *you will be better*).

IT'S NOT JUST FOOD . . . IT'S YOUR BRAIN

What helps protect our BRAINS?

- ✓ Low Sugar Intake (brains seems to like fat with normal amounts of blood sugar—not candy)
- ✓ Adequate Sleep
- ✓ Consuming Omega-3 (DHA)
- ✓ Good (high-density) Cholesterol
- ✓ Curcumin
- ✓ Regular Aerobic Exercise
- ✓ Occasional Fasting
- ✓ Regular Meals
- ✓ Following a Ketogenic Diet (numerous brain health studies)
- ✓ Decreasing Processed Grains

What can harm our brains?

- ✓ Eating Too Much Sugar
- ✓ Lack of Sleep
- ✓ Not Exercising
- ✓ Overeating

✓ High-Carbohydrate Diet/Grains (if you are sensitive)
✓ Too little *good* MUFA (monounsaturated fatty acids) Fats

A *slice* of bread is a slice of bread, right? Actually, no! A slice of whole rye bread is very different from a slice of refined rye or wheat bread. Whole rye is denser, higher in fiber, even has protein and does not have foamy fillers or dough softeners. And guess what else? It will not suddenly raise your blood sugar like refined flour does if you are sensitive to the carb-glucose conversion. A healthy slice of this "Roggen Brot," European whole kernel rye bread (available at health food stores and many markets) is delicious served with protein and fresh vegetables or slathered with creamy *real* butter and smoked salmon with dill, or even creamy nut butter and a teaspoon of fruit spread. Your body will let you know if what you are doing is working. For my diabetics, unfortunately even whole rye still affects their glucose—but that is not true for all of them. There are different levels of diabetes— whether one is insulin dependent or not. That is why it is *super important to personalize*

My 23 years of experience seeing 1000s of patients with chronic disease makes certain things quite obvious and one of them is that starchy and sugary carbohydrates seem to really aggravate certain health problems in diabetics and prediabetics. IF you are lean, healthy, have no diabetes in your family, have good appetite control, then this sensitivity may not seem realistic to you and that is okay. Learn from your body. That is why it is important to accept other people's journeys and physiological reactions to foods—as our chemistry, genetics and reactions to foods are all individualized—hence the science of nutrigenomics. As it sounds, it is based on Nutrition and Genetics . . .

and take what works for you from this book and **let go of what does not!**

Back to grains ... what about bread?

There is a difference between how we metabolize sugars and foods that turn to sugar. Realistically, most people will continue to eat bread, so it is helpful to choose the densest, most nutritious, least processed breads which are increasingly available in super markets, but if not, are always available at health food stores such as Trader Joe's, Whole Foods, Sprouts, etc. The price varies from $3.65 to $6.00, and are comparable to processed bread prices, unless you pick the cheapest white refined flour ones. In Southern and Northern California, particularly the coastal cities, chain supermarkets now offer true whole grain, (not "pretend whole grain" breads) as well as sprouted grain breads, like Ezekiel Bread—I know, not everyone's favorite, as it is chewier and denser. If you do not refrigerate Ezekiel, it can mold, especially in humid locations like the beautiful tropical Gulf Coast where I live. It may take some getting used to, but the great thing is that your energy and stamina will be noticeably improved and your hunger will be noticeably controlled when your foods contain more fiber. This of course does not work if you are whole-grain-sensitive or grain sensitive in general and certainly not if you are allergic, or have celiac disease etc. If so, then use the protein and vegetable options. Give healthy bread a try and see what works best for you. These breads are delicious with avocado, or a little bit of mayonnaise or Vegenaise®, hard-boiled egg and tomatoes or sliced cucumbers and dill with cream cheese or avocado toast spread. YUM! The natural fats from avocado and juices from the tomatoes, cucumbers and veggies add moisture to the true whole grain experience.

Differences Between Breads

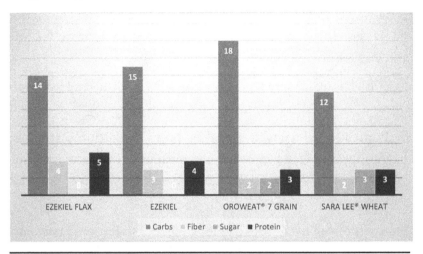

Figure 1: *Grams of carbohydrates, fiber, sugar and protein in different breads.*

A Quick Visual for You!

Bread	Carbs	Fiber	Sugar	Protein
Ezekiel Flax	14	4	0	5
Ezekiel	15	3	0	3
Oroweat® 7 grain	18	2	2	3
Sara Lee® wheat	12	2	3	3

Look at the actual ingredients and not just the nutrition facts. You should avoid fillers and additives like *corn-syrup*, *azodi-carbonamide* and avoid any unrecognizable words. (If you can't pronounce it—don't eat it) Compare sprouted bread with regular breads (be your own detective at the supermarket). More on this later! This was just a sneak peek! Over the last five years, since I started writing this book, bread manufacturers have begun to take away some of the chemical fillers, added synthetic flavorings and syrups. Consumer awareness and complaints spurred a movement for using *fresher, recognizable* ingredients.

Check Out These Funky Ingredients:

DATEM is an acronym for diacetyl tartaric acid esters of monoglycerides. This is a dough conditioner used to improve volume and uniformity in breads.

DATEM is considered safe by the FDA, but a study on rats showed "heart muscle fibrosis and adrenal overgrowth".[27]

Sodium stearoyl lactylates makes bread look fluffy. It is an FDA approved lactic acid-like chemical used in processed food, *but* it is *MORE PROCESSED* and *my point for you* is to eat *fresh* and *less processed* stuff.

Do you notice how a fresh baguette will get stale after a few days, maybe even one day? THAT'S GOOD! It was fresh and not filled with foamy, spongy additives. Yay, good, excellent—but if it stays fluffy for days, hmmm, you better remember that's not completely real in nature and this synthetic softener has been added to your food so you'll think it's fresh when it simply means this bread that lasts forever, or this icing that stays fluffy for days, has been processed more with fillers and synthetic goo . . . Keep it fresher, buy less, eat it and buy it again without all these funky fillers. (https://www.fooducate.com/product/Bimbo-Soft-White-Bread-Family/6589EEAE-E110-11DF-A102-FEFD45A4D471)

Eating your yoga mats? Almost!

The precursor to Yoga Mats, Vinyl and Foam: Azodicarbonamide is allowed to be added to flour at levels up to 45 parts per million (ppm) to condition flour for bread, or whiten cereal grains in the U.S. and Canada, but is banned in the European Union, Brazil, Australia and the United Kingdom. What if you eat more of these foods that contain this chemical . . . you can exceed the expected ppm intake and who knows what it's doing in your body. Logically, if it is not created by nature, the potential for aggravation in our body is greater. Even "naturally" occurring foods, or fresh foods can create allergic reactions or weird reactions like bloating, migraines, nausea, hives, etc. . . . adding a continuous barrage of synthetic foods can't possibly make you feel great in the long run! Thanks to Vani Hari of the Food Babe, recent use of it, has been slated to be removed and phased out in certain fast-food industries, check out her amazing website at www.foodbabe.com.

CHAPTER 6

The Food Balance Circus Act

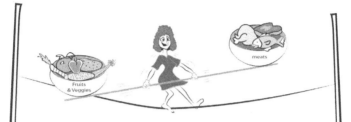

STEPS TO A HAPPY BODY: EAT FROM ALL TASTY FOOD GROUPS AND COLORS.

DO YOU FEEL like you are about to fall off that tight rope? You are not alone. Everyone has their ups and downs, their highs, their lows, but I am here to remind you that your intuition and keeping track of your personal inventory, will contribute to your healthier choices. If you feel better, you will continue. If you feel worse, you will reconsider. Do you want to get rid of those cravings and crazy hunger pangs? Not everyone has them, but a lot of us do and if you are struggling, look at the basics. Start with high soluble fiber (oats, oat bran, barley, apples) and lean protein, vegetables (have fiber and are low in sugar), whole grain such as wild rice (½ cup) or two sprouted grains, non-GMO (if that is even possible anymore) organic corn tortillas and make sure your plate is filled with a multitude of colors: green and yellow squash, carrots, ½ cup of black beans (if tolerated), three ounces of fish or chicken, one cup of baked yam with one tablespoon real butter or olive oil, spices, garlic, herbs and grilled onions. Fill it up, make it look great— fresh, clean, healthy, avoid all the pre-boxed, pre-cooked packed fast food low nutrient foods. Have some water and lime/ lemon, mint sprigs and enjoy. Dessert can be filled with poached pears dancing in cooked bourbon vanilla sauce or tangy honey citrus sauce or, indulge with dark chocolate squares and black berries . . . do not starve yourself.

What Do You Need?

✓ Eat one to two to three ounces of protein at each meal (palm of your hand) the more you weight the more you need—it can be vegetarian sourced.

✓ Protein—there are about seven grams of protein in one ounces of cooked meat, so three ounces furnishes about 21 grams. A typical 175-pound person needs about 50 to 64 grams of protein each day. This is only 1.7 to 2.2 ounces.

   • Options include lean meats, chicken, turkey, fish, egg, organic cottage cheese.

   • Vegan sources such as organic sprouted non-GMO tofu or soy (source matters), nuts: 25 walnuts provide about 15 grams, 1 cup cooked lentils provide 19 grams, 1 cup black beans provide 15.2 grams, 1 cup green peas provide 8 grams, 1 cup split peas provide 16 grams.

✓ Eat 1.5–2 cups of non-starchy vegetables at lunch and dinner and if you do that for breakfast you score.

✓ Eat ¾ to one cup of starch—quinoa, wild rice, yam, sweet potato, peas, sprouted grain.

✓ Occasional Basmati rice, or non-GMO pasta imported is fun from Italy.

- ✓ Eat one fruit, about one cup a day but avoid the juices.
- ✓ Avoid sugar drinks, juice, soda, processed bread as much as you can.
- ✓ Pick foods of different colors to get the benefit of all the plant pigments.
- ✓ Have a square of dark chocolate (helps reduce cortisol in some people).
- ✓ Use tasty oils—avocado, nuts, extra virgin olive oil at meals, helps absorb fat soluble vitamins such as Vitamin E and D, protects your organs and joints.
- ✓ Eat ½ cup legumes (if you are not sensitive to them and you are not avoiding lectins) three times per week— helps reduce risk of colon cancer, picks up cholesterol, helps to make your own probiotics (as veggies do) to protect your microbiome.
- ✓ Have 12 almonds or 7 walnuts, or one to two ounces nuts three to four times per week—helps decrease LDL oxidation, helps keep you full, gives you "good-for-you oils".
- ✓ Make sure to laugh every day!

WHAT YOU WILL EAT? YOUR GUIDE

Here are some fabulous selections Per Food Group:*

PROTEIN			
3 to 6 ounces per meal			
Red Meat	Poultry	Fish	Egg
Beef (1x week or less) Bison	Turkey Chicken All poultry	Salmon Sole Trout All Fish: Select lower mercury fish if you eat it over 3 times per week	Egg yolk/whites

NON-ANIMAL PROTEIN	
One ounce to two ounces per meal or day	
NUTS and SEEDS for ALL 3x per week	
NUTS (soaking them in water is good)	SEEDS
Walnuts Brazil Nuts Pecans (Eat less high lectin nuts such as: Cashews, peanuts) (Medium lectins: almonds)	Pumpkin Chia Sunflower Hemp Sesame Explore NON-GMO Organic sprouted Tofu (though controversy exists with soy)

NON-STARCHY VEGETABLES			
2 cups or more per plate			
Greens	Purples/Red	Orange/Yellow	White/Brown
Asparagus Artichoke Broccoli and Cabbage Celery and Endive Green beans Green Lettuce Green peppers (lectins; peel or moni- tor reaction) Kale and Spinach Swiss Chard Watercress Zucchini Fruit/ aka vegetable Avocado Cucumber	Beets (1/3 cup) Purple car- rots (sugary if cooked, raw is best) Pur- ple Cabbage Radicchio Radish Red Leaf Lettuce Red peppers (lectins; peel or moni- tor reaction)	Carrots (sugary if cooked, raw is best) Yellow pepper (lectins; peel or moni- tor reaction) Yellow Squash Butternut Squash	Cauliflower Garlic Mushrooms Onion (over cooked is too sweet; use more-raw or lightly cooked)

STARCHY VEGETABLES		
Use as starch vs. Grains if you wish		
½ cup to 1 cup (if you want to lose weight use less— listen to your body)		
Green	Yellow/Orange	White
Peas	Corn (try to find non-GMO or organic for reduced pesticide intake) Starchy squashes such as Butternut squash Sweet potato Yams	Cassava/Yuca/ Yucca root Parsnips Potatoes Turnips

GRAINS		
If you are grain sensitive avoid them		
Try to use non-GMO due to high pesticide and possible allergen reaction for SOME people		
1/2 cup—1 cup per plate vs starchy veg/or split the difference		
Rice or Hybrid Seed/Grain	Breads	Other/Crackers etc.
Brown Wild Basmati white (only ½ cup cooked; medium glycemic index, better than other white rice) Quinoa (high carb; measure it, it is not a "free food")	Sourdough (take it easy) (turns to sugar quickly 1 slice) Sprouted (turns to sugar slowly) Rye (100%) pumpernickel Rye mixed (5 ingredients) Pure without added sugar grains	Finn Crisps WASA crackers Rice crackers (gluten free) Mary's sprouted seed crackers (High Fiber)

Legumes

- If you are sensitive to beans and lentils, you can avoid them, please eat vegetables.
- ½ cup to 1 cup three times per week

- If you are using these as protein, you can increase to tolerance. There is conflicting evidence as to health risks and benefits.
- Make up your own mind. Monitor your physical reactions. I would say, keep balance, add them on occasion.

Fruit

- You can reduce fruit if you want to lose weight/control glucose/monitor reaction
- ½ to one cup if you have had one starch on the plate (reduce for weight loss)
- Low glycemic index (absorbs slower) (*) with low glycemic load (less total sugar)
- High glycemic index (**) low glycemic load (less total sugar)
- If you are diabetic, you may not tolerate fruit well: check your glucose (maximum glucose <180 2 hours post meals but prefer <141 glucose 2 hours post meals).

Green	Orange / Yellow	Purple / Blue
Green apple Green grapes** Honeydew Kiwi Limes* Tomato (high lectin; use ROMA or reduce, or peel or eat: monitor body reaction for arthritis/ or other)	Apricots Cantaloupe Crenshaw melon Lemon* Mango Nectarine Orange Papaya Peaches Persimmon Pineapple Tangerine Yellow Watermelon**	Blackberries* Blueberries* Concord grapes Plums Purple fig Watermelon

Red	White / Brown	
Blood orange Cherries Dried cranberries** Raw cranberries Pink grapefruit Pomegranates Raspberries* Red grapes** Red pears Strawberries Watermelon**	Banana ripe ** green/yellow * White peaches Dates** (very sweet it's a dessert have only one)	

Try new foods! Experiment.

Break the Routine

Your taste buds will love you when you create excitement in your mouth! That sounds rude, but seriously, if you eat the same thing, over-and-over again, it is less likely for you to eat well. Eating well is NOT eating boring food, it is eating from the earth—real foods that grow from the ground and trees and come from the sea (if you are not vegetarian). TRY recipes from new countries, try new flavors, try new condiments and spices, take a risk with a new spice.

If you do not want to cook, there are premade salads and fresh cooked foods at stores, not the Frozen meals, but the fresh cooked meals. When you look at the food you will KNOW if it has the healthy protein, vegetables and starch in it, or if it is all processed.

If you do like to cook, you can have fresh new recipes through meal prep delivery boxes with incredibly diverse spices such as Thai, Indian, Italian, Moroccan and any other variety of deliciousness. Here are some great meal box delivery services: Hello Fresh, Home Chef, Freshly (Gluten Free options), Home Chef Fresh and Easy and Veestro (Vegan options). These have excellent directions and new ways of using herbs, spices and flavors so you will not get bored.

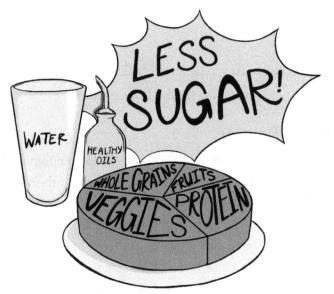

Artist credit: Lindy Plunkett (made for Dr. Dani, Ph.D.)

CHAPTER 7

Intermittent Fasting

Kick Start Fat burning and Regenerate Your Cells

Note: Please do not do this if you have had a diagnosis of having an eating disorder. Thank you.

ALWAYS CONSULT WITH YOUR PRIMARY CARE PROVIDER

IT'S TRUE! INTERMITTENT fasting has been shown in numerous peer reviewed science and medical journals to WORK. What does it do? Among many things, two outstanding metabolic effects are:

It helps you burn fat stores.

It helps regenerate your cells.

The longer the fasting period past 16 hours, the more detox happens to help you regenerate cells and burn fat

12-16-24 HOUR FASTS—DRINK PLENTY OF WATER

Twelve Hour Fast

Twelve hours of fasting daily should be the minimum to allow your body to begin dealing with stored toxins, fats and to help improve digestion. Keeping the same 12-hour window might be a good start to adhere to a routine. Keep it the same every day.

For example, seven a.m. to seven p.m. daily, or nine a.m. to nine p.m. daily. Drink water—**HALF OF YOUR WEIGHT IN OUNCES, OR ABOUT 2.5 LITERS IS A SAFE BET.**

Sixteen Hour Fast

Sixteen hours of not eating, with an eight-hour window of eating normal meals (not the whole time) have been shown to improve digestion and help with appetite control.

You can try this once a week, or daily, or any amount of days you want. Make sure your meals are nutritious, healthy and do not eat fast food or processed packaged foods as you are working on cleaning house! It's logical that if you give your 21-28 feet of intestines a rest, a bit of regeneration can occur. That goes for all your accessory organs, which are your pancreas, liver and gall-bladder. They a need a vacation too.

Twenty-four Hour Fast

Twenty-four hours of fasting, with water and about 500 calories of broth—natural not canned, is a great break through fast, after you've broken into the 12 to 18 hour one. Avoid anything with syrups and sugars (consult your doctor). Drink 2.5 liters of water or drink half of your body weight in pounds, in ounces. For example: If you weigh 200 pounds, you would drink 100 ounces of water. If you sweat, or exercise, drink an additional 8 to 16 ounces per thirty minutes of sweating. If you live in the tropics and you sweat all day, keep drinking eight or more ounces per hour to replenish your stores of water, along with electrolytes, sodium and potassium. Add broth and vegetable juices—home pressed to about 500 calories per day.

Try this anywhere from once a week, twice a week, or up to three days. Consult your primary healthcare provider.

Twelve hours can also help you, but it has less effect on stored fat. However, all the hours of rest from digesting foods 2-4-7 allows your body to get rid of stored toxins—instead of working on digestion in your gut, the body has a chance to clean its cells—as hours increase to 24 hours, then apoptosis increases. What is apoptosis? It is cell death and great to get rid of unwanted cells—like cleaning your closet and throwing out old shoes. It also allows your digestive system to work on getting rid of stored junk and gives the body a break from constantly digesting what you are giving it.

Sixteen hours of fasting can begin the process of fat burning, which releases the fat stores into your blood stream, which in turn provides **Ketones** (energy from fat in your blood). Some studies suggest ten hours can begin this process, especially for those who have never fasted before. The more hours, the more results, according to scientific literature.[28]

If you fast, but consume liquor, you might not see much of a weight loss change as that liquor stores as fat.

Just like going through an automatic car wash, cells do a **Self Cell Wash** when you fast. Even 12 hours of fasting can initiate that process. This **Self-Cleaning** is called autophagy. When we give our bodies rest from digesting our masses of delicious food intake, it has an opportunity to clean old gunk and junk from our cells. If it is too busy working on what we are putting in, then it does not get a chance to clean itself. IF we are too busy with other things, the organization and cleaning flies out the window.

A wonderful *Netflix* reality show called Tidying UP with Mari Kondo, Japanese lifestyle guru sensation, (https://www.netflix.com/title/80209379), transforms lives and relationships by the power of tidying up. Mari calls these magical results a form to **spark joy**, our cells need a little **spark joy** vibe too.

Do you want improved health and lifespan? Improve glucose metabolism!

Research in animal studies demonstrate improved live span and improved health with intermittent fasting.[29] In humans, we see disease reduction as a result of intermittent fasting, even though in humans it is difficult to maintain.[30] However, for those who do, the benefits include a decrease in **Metabolic Syndrome**. Metabolic syndrome is also known as insulin resistance and is associated with the following conditions: glucose intolerance, upper body fat distribution (ab fat), hypertension (high blood pressure), dysfibrinolysis (blood clotting issues), dyslipidemia (high triglycerides), low good cholesterol (HDL), bad LDL increases, proinflammation occurs and clotting is influenced as well.[31] The risks are all over the place from heart disease, to diabetes and inflammatory disorders. **However**, intermittent fasting seems to help minimize these.

Can I do Intermittent Fasting if I am diabetic?

YES: But you must monitor your blood glucose and adjust your medication and insulin according to your doctor's guidance as you will have longer periods of not eating. Make sure to talk to your primary care provider. Good results have been seen in insulin sensitivity (*your* insulin works better). Review these hyperlinks if you are interested: https://www.mdpi.com/2077-0383/8/10/1645/htm and https://www.nia.nih.gov/news/research-intermittent-fasting-shows-health-benefits.

You can also always keep up with NIH updates and you can easily use google scholar and type in intermittent fasting and obesity, or any other topic you want to tackle, such as diabetes, or insulin use, etc.

CHAPTER **8**

Six Cups of Sugar Per Week

WELCOME TO THE WORLD OF SUGAR AND SWEETENERS!

Centers for Disease Control (CDC), Soda, Fat, US and the World

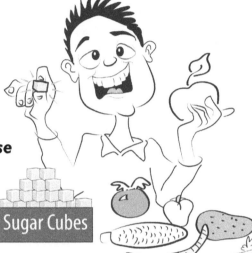

Sugar Cubes

APPROXIMATELY 50% OF the US population consume sugar drinks (does not include 100% fruit juice or diet drinks) and about 10% consume three or more sugar drinks per day. Canadians also consume at least 19.7 ounces per day of sugar drinks, with Australians reportedly consuming 14 to 22 teaspoons of added sugars per day. Recently the CDC reported information: that 67% of the US population drinks daily sodas! There is a variation in states and demographic breakdown, with Mississippi leading at 41% of the population reporting at least sweet drink per day, followed by Tennessee, Nevada, Oklahoma and Georgia. That does not include sugary coffees and the new multi teaspoon syrup pump craze. Additional information indicates that six in ten kids in the US and five in ten adults drink sweetened beverages. The Harvard School of Public

Health, CDC and scientific literature concur that the increase in sugar beverages is correlated with the increase in childhood and adult obesity.

WORLD WIDE SUGAR CONSUMPTION

Year / Country	Sugar Consumption
1600s: United Kingdom	7 pounds/year/person
1850s: United States	52 pounds/year/person
1970s: United States	125 pounds/year/person
2003: United States	150 pounds/year/person
2014: United States	42.5 TABLESPOON per day (DHHS)
2020: United States	6 cups per week, 152 pounds per year/person
12 ounces Pepsi	9-11.7 teaspoons
12 ounces Coke	9-12 teaspoons
Since 1974: sugar intake	Doubled
Since 1942: soda intake	Increased 7-fold

Sugar drink sales around the world show us that the US is not the only one in trouble when it comes to excess sugar drink intake. Chile and Mexico lead the way above the U.S., but all the rest follow: Argentina, Saudi Arabia, Germany, Netherlands, Slovakia, Austria and Brazil. (https://www.cdc.gov/nchs/products /databriefs/db71.htm)

If we ate more *whole* foods instead of liquid sugars and processed foods, we would likely feel better and in the long run, have fewer health issues:

Fructose and **Glucose**: Calories and Health Risks

What are the relations between sugar consumption and becoming overweight or obese?

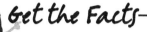

Get the Facts

2020 CDC data—Behavioral Issues and Sugar Drinks

Here is a direct quote from the CDC's website on sugar consumption, including sugar-sweetened-beverages (SSBs)

"SB consumption is associated with less healthy behaviors.

Adults and adolescents who smoke, don't get enough sleep, don't exercise much, eat fast food often and who do not eat fruit regularly are more likely to be frequent consumers of SSBs. Additionally, adolescents who frequently drink SSBs also have more screen time (e.g., television, cell phones, computers, video games)."

You can find the data in this link: https://www.cdc.gov/nutrition/data-statistics/sugar-sweetened-beverages-intake.html

Sugar Consumption in USA

I gallon of sugar = 768 teaspoons

Americans consume 15% of their daily calories from sugars

152 pounds of annual sugar consumption equals six cups of sugar per week.

An international study involving 128 countries showed a relationship among sugar intake, cereal intake; and less physical activity increased obesity risk. The study was not "linear," meaning it does not state that everyone who doesn't exercise or who eats sugar and cereal has weight problems. It merely looked at thousands of people to find associations and correlations between what they were doing and what their health outcomes were. Statistically, those who did little physical activity and ate sugar and cereals weighed more than those who did not.

> **National Center of Health Statistics**
>
> Children consume 1,000–2,000 calories from soda per day. This increases risk of fatty liver, heart disease, obesity, kidney issues, cavities and diabetes.
>
> Refined sugar comprises 15% of the U.S. calorie consumption.

The American Heart Association recommends less than nine teaspoons per day for men, less than six teaspoons per day for women and less than 100 calories per day from added sugars.

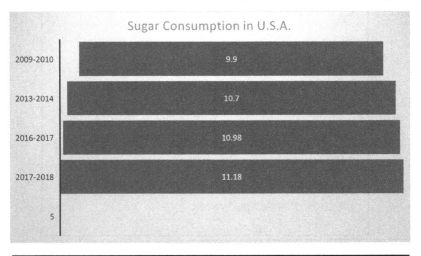

Figure 2: *Adapted from Statista Agricultural Statistics in million metric tons (https://www.statista.com/statistics/249692/us-sugar-consumption/)*

Each teaspoon of sugar contains fifteen calories (nine teaspoons times fifteen calories = 135 calories). It is recommended that you obtain less than ten percent of your calories from sugar. If you eat 1,800 calories you should not have more than 180 calories from all sugars.

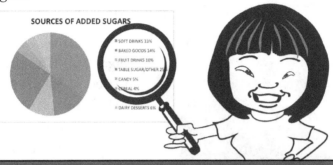

SOURCES OF ADDED SUGARS

- SOFT DRINKS 33%
- BAKED GOODS 14%
- FRUIT DRINKS 10%
- TABLE SUGAR/OTHER 25%
- CANDY 5%
- CEREAL 4%
- DAIRY DESSERTS 6%

THE AKA'S OF SUGAR
I Spy More Sneaky Sugar!

Sugar Brown, White, Powdered	Fruit fresh is good— careful with large smoothies and juices **too much** fructose can increase weight	**Note:** Fruit juice has more sugar than soda Grape juice has more than Sprite! Neither are helpful to your weight goals!	Grape juice: 150 calories and 36 grams carbs
All Syrup	Molasses / Honey	Isomalt	Dextrin and HSH: hydro-genated starch hydrosolates
Beet sugar	Maltodextrin	Corn syrup	
Fruit Juice Concentrate	High fructose Corn Syrup Any "ose" ending Lactose Maltose Dextrose Glucose Fructose	Sorghum syrup "itol" endings are sugar alcohols used in sugar-free stuff Erythritol Lactitol (from milk) Maltitol Mannitol Sorbitol Xylitol (ok)	Corn Sweetener Agave (20–30% sweeter than sugar) Up to 93% fructose

HOW MANY METRIC TONS OF SUGAR ARE CONSUMED IN THE US?

From 2017 to 2018 **11.18 million metric tons of sugar were consumed in the U.S.** A difference of 1.2 million metric tons from 2009 to 2017.

11.8 MILLON METRIC TON OF SUGAR

USA

Sugar Consumption in the U.S. in Million Metric Tons Expected Sugar intake by 2023 is 13 million metric tons. World Sugar Production 2020 is 165.8 Million metric tons.

How many calories do you get from sugar?

You may be consuming more calories from sugar than you know. One teaspoon of white sugar gives you 15 calories. One teaspoon of corn syrup or honey gives you 20 calories. If a can of soda has

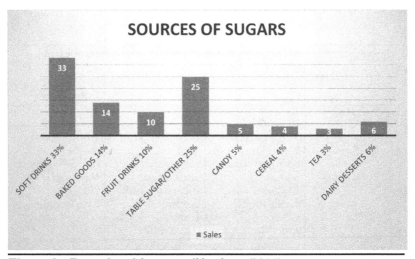

SOURCES OF SUGARS

33 — SOFT DRINKS 33%
14 — BAKED GOODS 14%
10 — FRUIT DRINKS 10%
25 — TABLE SUGAR/OTHER 25%
5 — CANDY 5%
4 — CEREAL 4%
3 — TEA 3%
6 — DAIRY DESSERTS 6%

■ Sales

Figure 3: *Data adapted from www.dhhs.nh.gov (2014)*
Note: Main source of sugar comes from soda

12 teaspoons of corn syrup, on average, how many calories are in one 8 ounce can of soda? **Answer:** 240 calories. If you are drinking a fountain drink from a soda dispenser, you may have a variable dose of sugar because the level of syrup added may not be mea-

> **Calories from Sugar**
>
> - 1 tsp. white sugar: 15 calories
> - 1 tsp. honey: 20 calories
> - 1 tsp. corn syrup: 20 calories
> - 1 tsp. molasses: 22 calories

sured properly. The amount of ice you use also changes the total calories as you may have more ice than soda. If you want 100% fruit juice, be aware that eight ounces of fresh juice also contains high amounts of fructose and some fruit juices have added corn syrup, so try to avoid juice. Excess amounts of fructose, depending on your needs, can keep you from losing stored fat and may contribute to storing even more fat.

ARTIFICIAL SWEETENERS

Aspartame, newly named *AminoSweet*, is an artificial sweetener that is 200 times sweeter than sugar. It has been the source of much scientific and consumer debate. Financially it has cost companies and consumers $570 million and counting annually.[32] To some, it is a serious concern. In animal studies, the sweetener has demonstrated tumor growth and neurological damage. Many people have reactions like headaches, nausea, joint pain, vision problems and vomiting. I have never tolerated artificial sweeteners. When aspartame came out in the 1980s, I had no idea it existed in my foods. I did not know anything about the harsh side effects. I tried a breath mint and got sick. When I read the ingredients, although at the time I had no understanding, but noted the personal havoc. Then I had a piece of gum. I got nauseous and developed a headache. I read the ingredients again. This time,

I recognized the word "aspartame" and knew I probably should avoid aspartame. Years later, I tried a friend's candy and got sick again. There it was again. My lesson was very clear, I need to stay away from aspartame. Not everyone reacts physically or is aware of the cause of their inflammatory reaction to aspartame. You are chemically different and may not react the same way I do. Studies demonstrate some people are more susceptible to headaches when ingesting aspartame (https://n.neurology.org /content/44/10/1787.short; and https://www.researchgate.net /profile/Prof_Shrivastava/publication/316545292_Aspartame _Effects_and_Awareness/links/590311660f7e9bcf654b2370 /Aspartame-Effects-and-Awareness.pdf).

What is aspartame? Oh my, storing bodies in formaldehyde. What!? This is what it is if you want more information, aspartame is a dipeptide of two amino acids ("di" for two): aspartic acid and phenylalanine. It breaks down into formaldehyde—so do fruits and jelly beans, which makes the formaldehyde argument with aspartame difficult to win. However, aspartame breaks down into more substances such as phenylalanine, methanol and aspartic acid. Each of these, in excessive amounts, have caused neurologic and brain problems in animal studies.[33] Multiple animal studies demonstrate side effects with high levels of aspartame, unlike effects from high fruit intake.

In my opinion, it is unnecessary to use a synthetic additive when there are less toxic options available such as xylitol or stevia (pure form). Better yet, just skip it altogether! However, several proponents of aspartame, including the American Cancer Society (www.cancer.org), propose that since the FDA has "approved" the use of aspartame, it should be considered generally safe.[34] Unfortunately, as more and more products include aspartame (aka: "AminoSweet") the number of people consuming the products daily is on the rise. *There is a rumor that milk will include aspartame without being labeled as having aspartame.* It is important that consumers are aware which products have aspartame as there is an upper limit of safety. If every diet product contains aspartame, it is possible to exceed the upper limit. Over time, the risks increase.

The European Food Safety Authority (EFSA) sets the upper limit of aspartame intake for humans at 40 micrograms/kilograms (40 micrograms/2.2 pounds) of your weight. The U.S. FDA sets the upper limit at 50 micrograms/kilograms. One can of diet soda contains 1.2 grams (1,200 micrograms.) of aspartame. If you weigh 150 pounds, your upper limit of aspartame intake should be less than 2,700 micrograms.

I had a client who drank two liters of diet coke a day. He weighed about 190 pounds, which made his upper limit 3,450 micrograms. He was drinking approximately 10,140 micrograms of aspartame NutraSweet® or Equal® per day. We cannot attribute my patient's health issues directly to aspartame, but he continuously complained of weight problems, bloating, inflammation, depression, fatigue and eventually died (at age 55) in his sleep. Research is ongoing in animal studies regarding tumors, cancers and aspartame.[35,36] The accumulation over many years may cause unknown health risks, much like those seen in rat studies. The results are seen in Dr. Soffriti's seven-year animal aspartame study. Dr. Soffriti is a cancer researcher and scientific director of the non-profit European Ramazzini Foundation of Oncology cancer research organization.[37] Hyperlinks provided by the NIH (National Institute of Health) on Dr. Soffriti's work were originally available when I researched the data but were later not available anymore a few months later. It is curious to me that it should have been eliminated from the NIH database, though I am hopeful they will have it available soon, so that I may share the results with you. Alas, in 2021 I found the rebuttal letter from

2008 by Dr. Soffriti and the explanation of the scholarly battering he got from colleagues when he published concerns about aspartame. Here you go: https://www.ncbi.nlm.nih.gov/pmc/articles/PMC2430255/

Some physicians are concerned of potential blood-brain barrier destruction by aspartame, associated with excessive glutamate in the brain. The condition possibly increases Alzheimer's risks. There are no conclusive studies in humans. Aspartame was originally *not approved* by the FDA but later "approved" under what some suspect were controversial practices. Some of the reported side effects of Aspartame are headaches, abdominal weight gain, diabetes risk and multiple sclerosis-like symptoms in some people, which disappear after consumption is discontinued. Multiple Sclerosis (MS) symptoms does not mean having MS, it just means some people have physiological reactions that are similar to MS if they react adversely to aspartame (though it is rare). The good news is that if aspartame is causing neurological problems, it can be reversed once you stop drinking or eating aspartame containing foods.

SUGAR, FRUCTOSE, FAT STORAGE, AND INFLAMMATION

SNEAKY SOURCES OF SUGAR MAY SURPRISE YOU!

SOURCES OF HIDDEN CORN SYRUP BEWARE

We've all grown up hearing, "Eat fruit, it's good for you!" or "If it's a fruit shake, that's a healthy choice." When I ask my patients what they've been eating, invariably their diet will include several servings of fructose-rich meals, not only from multiple servings of fruit (even whole, fresh fruit) but from high-fructose corn syrup (corn syrup comes from corn and is highly processed and concentrated), grains and other *sneaky sugar* foods such as:

Sneaky Sugars:

Pasta Sauces jarred	Salad Dressing	Pre-made Dough
(look at ingredients =	Some spices, salts,	Breads and
avoid added syrup . . .)	flavorings	Wheat Bread
Crackers	Fruit Drinks	Breath Mint
Gum,	Cereals	Deli Meat
Candy,	Flavored Yogurt	Frozen Dinners
Chocolate	Processed Foods	Bagels
Canned Fruit	Sports or Health Drink	

A little bit of these foods with sneaky sources of sugar is perfectly fine and can be metabolized by your body, but an accumulation of fructose causes a chemical reaction in your fat cells to store more fat. Often you just don't seem to know *why* you don't feel full. You keep eating to satisfy hunger, causing the weight gain to continue. When this occurs, fat loss through burning stored fat for energy does not occur. At the end of the day, you may be consuming 20 times more corn syrup than you are aware of without ever having added one teaspoon of sugar! This is a contemporary problem—too much fructose and sugars in too many places. This leads to discouragement and frustration on your part or just plain giving up. Here is an example of a patient who was unaware of how much corn syrup he was consuming:

Bagel from popular chain uses corn syrup in their dough; oatmeal sweetened with corn syrup; juice and sports drink daily sweetened with corn syrup; crackers saying wheat contained no fiber but were loaded with sugar and corn syrup; snack bar with what he thought were whole grains contained 27 grams of sugar mainly from corn syrup; fancy coffee with two pumps of flavoring was made of pure corn syrup; ready-made pasta sauce with spaghetti and a soda. By the end of the day he had corn syrup with every meal and every snack and he didn't even know it. Ask yourself if you are like this man.

*You are sabotaging fat loss with corn syrup in sodas and sweet
drinks. Too many people are not aware of how these liquids
can alter their body's capacity to burn and use fat and sugar.*

Everyone's chemical composition is unique. These differences
reflect how and what changes you must make in your dietary
intake and physical activity levels. Some people can eat more fruit
and grains than others. You get to choose what works best for
you based on your individual body chemistry. I will simply give
you the facts to help you make informed choices. In my practice,
women over 40 who are not physically active (especially menopausal and post-menopausal women) do not lose weight easily
when consuming more than two cups of fruit a day (especially
when they are also eating grains). They need to balance the two.
Unless they consume meals that consist of lean protein and vegetables, and they avoid juice or sugar beverages, they often struggle
to lose or maintain weigh loss. They are very active and work on
muscle tone and strength. The balance between the total amount
of glucose converting carbohydrates is crucial. A balance between
starches and fruits is important, and on the days where more fruit
is eaten, less starchy foods should be consumed. Think of balanc-
ing the scales.

You may do better without fruit for a few weeks, or two weeks,
as recommend by Dr. David Perlmutter, MD. Then you can add
back low-glycemic index fruits such as berries, then gradually add
other fruits (not in juice form as that sugar absorbs too quickly).
The more active you are, the more you're able to burn those extra
fructose calories. It's extremely personalized! Everybody is different. The more you exercise, the more you burn. The better you
metabolize blood glucose, the more you can consume fruit and
some grains. You must keep track of how you respond. It's really
about the balance of your whole day. Fruit is healthy, find the
amount that works for you. By the way, skipping fruit as a test

for two weeks doesn't mean you are carbohydrate loading with bagels and processed breads or cereals. That won't work either. Here is the logical approach: Healthy meal, a few days or two weeks without fruit as an experiment and then add the fruit back into your day and observe and chart how you feel. How you feel includes how your body feels: bloated, light, heavier, fatigued, energized, hungry, or satisfied.

Remember, fructose in fruit is sweet and triggers certain enzymes in your cells to store fat. The nutrients in fruits are important, but you must figure out what works for your unique metabolism. If you eat well and include fruit in your diet with regular exercise consisting of 150 to 300 minutes per week and you are happy with your weight, energy and health, that's excellent! *Do what works for you.* You can start slowly and test different fruits for a few days. Balance is essential . . . not only with food but with your emotional and spiritual state. To monitor your daily progress, I suggest keeping track of what you eat and how you feel in a journal.

Exercise is recommended by the American Heart Association and the National Cancer Institute as well as the Diabetes Association, but you can lose weight without lots of exercise if you eat only what your body requires. I am not recommending a *no exercise* life style . . . . there are so many benefits to exercise. I am suggesting you find a happy way to incorporate a few minutes a day of physical activity and keep adding *fun* activities, so you don't feel like you are punishing yourself with forced exercise. Do what you love and what inspires you. Some people need more exercise than others, so be sure not to judge your friends who exercise a lot to keep weight in check just because you don't need to exercise as much. PS, vice versa too! As a human, you love being right; but *it's a lot more fun to be around cheerleaders than around know-it-alls!*

SUGARS=URIC ACID = INFLAMMATION

Have you ever heard of uric acid? High sugar intake is associated with elevated levels of uric acid which can lead to gout. Gout is the diagnosis where uric acid creates a painful, crystal-like substance which gets stuck in your joints like shards of glass. Gout also occurs in people who cannot process purines (protein metabolism by-products) from proteins such as red meat, chicken, beans and even nuts. I have never had a patient with gout who was vegetarian or vegan. Most of my gout patients over the last 18 years have been males with a high intake of meats and a low intake of vegetables. The patients tend to consume soda or sugary drinks much more than water throughout the week. Some of my gout patients weren't eating vegetables at all but had a high meat, soda, or alcohol consumption.

Vegans, Vegetarians, Meat Eaters and Gout

An interesting study about uric acid levels and food consumption patterns comparing vegetarians, vegans, fish eaters and meat eaters provided surprising results. Vegans had the highest concentration of serum uric acid levels, followed by meat eaters . . . but the lowest concentrations of uric acid was found in vegetarians and fish eaters.[38] You would think that since vegans consume purine-rich raw seeds, cauliflower and beans they would have **more** gout symptoms (that painful joint pain in the big toe or knee which swells up, is red and hurt like the dickens!) But that was not the case. This vegan diet may have provided some sort of protection against gout. Generally speaking, it's best to consume less red meat and pork and increase fish and plant-based foods to maintain appropriate uric acid and pH levels. Go plants!

Get the Facts
Wild Facts about Depression and Uric Acid

What about people diagnosed with depression? Do they have high uric acid levels?

While conducting research, I was surprised to discover that people with depression actually had uric acid levels that were too low, but teens diagnosed with depression had high levels, as did those diagnosed with bi-polar disorder or schizophrenia!

For those with depression, their levels stabilized once they took anti-depressants. Why am I bringing this up? Because we are intricately connected internally; we are a mass of chemicals thrown together in a miraculous way and the balance of all our nutrients which affect our chemistry is extremely important. Not only do uric acid levels reflect psychiatric states, but high uric acid wreaks havoc on the body causing excruciating pain and destroying tissue. Most importantly, it is extremely damaging to your cardiovascular system.

What's my point? All things in balance! Have some vegetables if you like meat and explore alternatives, different portions. Listen to your body and your mind. There is no better watchdog than yourself.

CHAPTER **9**

Weight and Your Health

What is YOUR healthy weight?

DON'T THINK SKINNY. That's not what we are talking about. Don't even think athletic, or low body fat. That's not it either. Healthy weight means you are at the weight where the increased risk of weight related diseases is reduced, for a healthier life. What are these risks that you reduce with healthy weight? Diabetes risk is reduced with healthy weight, as there is a positive correlation (as one changes so does the other) between increased weight and increased diabetes risk. More and more people without any relatives with diabetes are developing diabetes and more and more people are overweight or obese. What's going on?

You probably know when your own weight (due to fat, not muscle) is higher than it should be to maintain optimal health, regardless of the BMI results. Healthy weight is considered having a BMI of less than 25. However, if you are a body builder and are very muscular, or built with denser bones and higher muscle mass, the results need to be adjusted. Ethnicity and overall body composition can also affect BMI. I don't want you to only focus on BMI (unless your BMI is above 35, as those numbers don't always take into account your bone density, lean body mass (muscle mass) and ethnicity). A BMI of 35 already has an increased risk of health issues. But you can start navigating towards a BMI closer to 25, little-by-little, as you stay active and eat well without dieting or starving! A better way to see how your weight is doing is to measure the inches around your waist, which I will be explaining in the next section.

How many inches increase YOUR Risk for Heart Disease and Diabetes?

Males with waist circumference of 37 inches are at risk, with 40 inches increasing diabetes and heart disease risk. Females with waist circumference of 31.5 inches are at risk, with 35 inches increasing diabetes and heart diseases risk.

BMI is measured by using your weight in kilograms and dividing it by your height in meters squared [kilograms divided by meters squared] you can also do it through conversion web-sites: get my BMI through the NIH website. You can google "get my BMI" or go to NIH link: https:// www.nhlbi.nih.gov/health/educational /lose_wt/BMI/bmicalc .htm. Let's look at what is BMI ranges below:

- ✓ BMI less than 25 is healthy
- ✓ BMI of 25 - 29.99 is overweight
- ✓ BMI of 30 - 35 is obese
- ✓ BMI above 35 has an obesity grade of I or II; above 40 "morbid" obesity

Waist Circumference

Waist circumference is the inches measured around your waist. It even more important than BMI (if your BMI is less than 35). The total inches around your waist are associated with higher risk of health issues like diabetes. Health risks are what you want to reduce and eliminate to the best of your ability. *Waist Circumference is the most important thing related to disease risk!*

The Heart Issue with a Fatty Belly?

A little fat around the belly as we get older is normal, but once that spare tire around your waist gets bigger and bigger, it is a sure sign that you are eating more than your body can burn, especially sugar and fructose (sugar from fruit or corn syrup). I must admit, the yogis I have met who are in their 60s do *not* have rolls of fat around their bellies. When I saw my 58-year-old friend, Sheldon L, looking as lean as when I first met him 26 years ago, I remembered that he is a yoga practitioner—breathing and doing yoga

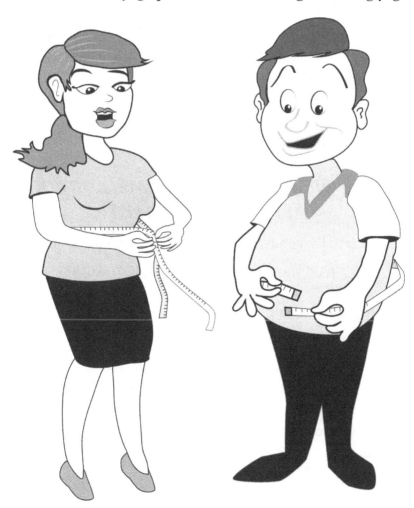

daily for at least two hours every day. Sheldon eats very healthy unprocessed foods, does not drink alcohol, avoids wheat and dairy and does not consume sugars (except some fruits). He is quite remarkable and seemingly ageless as he travels the world holding yoga seminars and teaching others. Often it is said that weight gain will occur with age. However, healthy lifestyle can maintain longevity and a positive body at any age (barring thyroid or medical issues). My friend's healthy, "lean and clean" meals, as well as his regular meditation, exercise and breathing exercises improved his health, vitality and youthful appearance.

This lifestyle is supported by Dr. Dean Ornish's treatment methodology. As a result, he documented improved cardiovascular recovery rates in his medical practice by encouraging meditation, low-fat meals, plant-based foods and sleep. Dr. Ornish's success rate in patient recovery from heart disease is high and well-respected in the medical community.[39]

HOW 'WEIRD FOOD' RECOMMENDATIONS AFFECT YOUR WEIGHT!

Lists, Pyramids, Circles and Plates Oh my! What?

Wild Recommendations from 1917–2018!

Trivia of Recommendations

There have been all kinds of incarnations of "what to eat" from the squares and circles, to the pyramid and now the healthy plate!

The first food recommendations in the U.S. in 1894 provided a 30-page document of guidelines. From 1917 through the 1920s, basic "How to select foods" were recommended to both children and adults, but by 1941 the RDA (recommended daily allowance) was created and created the Daily 7.

The Daily 7: 7 Food Groups in the form of a wheel specifying different colored fruits and vegetables, proteins and fats: 1) green and yellow veggies (raw, cooked, frouncesen, canned); 2) oranges, tomatoes, grapefruit, raw cabbage, salad greens; 3) potatoes and other veggies, fruits, raw, dried, cooked, frouncesen, canned; 4) milk and milk products; 5) meat, poultry, fish, eggs, dried beans, peas, nuts; 6) bread, cereal, flour, whole grain, enriched, restored; 7) butter or fortified margarine with added Vitamin A. They were more spe-

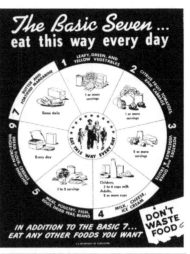

Figure 4: *By U.S. Department of Agriculture - 20111110-OC-AMW-0012\, Public Domain, https://commons.wikimedia.org/w/index.php?curid=17794846*

cific then and apparently people were annoyed as it was "too complex," so the "Basic Four" was created.

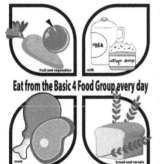

The Basic Four: 1) vegetables and fruits; 2) milk; 3) meat; 4) cereals and breads. By the 1970s, people were eating way too much disease-causing food groups, as the **Basic Four** gave equal importance to all food groups, which provided too much saturated fat from dairy and meat and processed grains, sugars and not enough produce. You can imagine the upheaval of the meat and dairy industry. By 1979, a *fifth* group was created to help reduce the intake of total fats, sweets and alcohol.

In 1984 a **new approach** included the "**Food Wheel:** A Pattern for Daily Food Choices" with **five** mayor food groups.

The "Food Pyramid" showed up in the 1990s, but its formation (types of foods in the food pyramid) was heavily lobbied by food companies and provided a skewed excess focused on grains. After much controversial lobbying, it was presented to the U.S. public, followed for a bit, recognized as too heavy in grains and then modified by Harvard Health Publications to The Healthy Eating Pyramid which had much less grain though it included whole food grains and large amounts of vegetables and fruits, healthy good oils/fats and exercise as part of a healthy lifestyle. The 1992 recommended six to eleven daily servings of bread, cereal, rice and pasta proved to be way too much for the average person!

Gradually, in 2011, U.S., First Lady, Michelle Obama and the Agriculture Secretary, Tom Vislack, announced the new guidelines; the building of a "**Healthy Plate**".

Now, we have www.ChooseMyPlate.gov, which depicts a healthy plate divided into 50% fruits and vegetables, approximately 25% each of lean protein and whole grains, a side of dairy and water vs. sweet drinks.

The original 1940s seven food group specified the colors of produce and if it hadn't been simplified to the 4 food groups, we may have had a better U.S. diet in the last 7 to 8 decades. Again, that produce is important!

OVERWEIGHT AND OBESITY

In my practice while counseling people on nutrition, I often see the horrified look in my patients' eyes when they catch a glimpse of the Electronic Medical Record (EMR) which automatically calculates BMI (Body Mass Index) and provides a diagnosis: morbid obesity, or obesity.

This is disconcerting, to say the least and the words "obese" or "morbidly obese" are psychologically disturbing. I have had patients receive an official diagnosis of "OBESE" from a calculation that did not account for their more than average lean body mass and their high bone density.

Your body is unique and individual! Please don't focus on these words or labels. These are not useful and should only be used as medical codes for medical tracking purposes. The objective is to find your healthy weight and happily *navigate* a combination of choices that allow for vibrant energy, deep sleep, a strong immune system and longevity!

ACCORDING TO WHO(M)? THE WORLD HEALTH ORGANIZATION

The world is suffering from an increased prevalence of obesity with the World Health Organization (WHO) reporting over 1.4 billion adults 20 and older as overweight and over 600 million men and women as obese. I will provide you with U.S. and international statistics and weight limits as they are associated with increased risk of diabetes, cardiovascular disease, joint issues, depression, hormonal imbalances and increased risk of cancer. These are just for your information: Think of it as health trivia!

- Worldwide obesity has nearly doubled since 1980.
- More than 40 million children under the age of five were overweight in 2011.
- In 2008 more than 1.4 billion adults (20 and over) were overweight; 200 million men and nearly 300 million women were obese.
- Thirty-five percent of adults (20 and over) were overweight in 2008; 11% were obese.
- In the U.S. adult population 42.4% are obese, an increase of 26% since 2008.

- Sixty five percent of the world's population lives in countries where overweight and obesity kills more people than those that are underweight.
- Obesity is often preventable! Its severity is manageable, no matter what your genetics!

How many people are overweight in the U.S.?

The numbers are astounding: 62% of the United States population is overweight. Our **2020 data confirms that over 40% of US adults are obese.** This figure is over twice as high as in 1960 (National Center for Health Statistics). Because having weight issues increases risk of disease, it is vital to take seriously the importance of regaining health and well-being.

SURPRISING WEIGHT STATS IN THE U.S. 2014

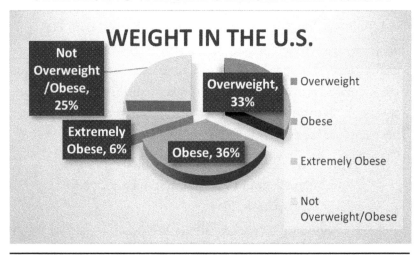

Figure 5: *Adopted from National U.S. Statistics percent prevalence of overweight and obesity in the U.S. (The National Institute of Health, 2014): 33.1% of adults are overweight; 35.7% are obese; 6.4% are extremely obese. Approximate percentage of healthy weight in the U.S. is 24.8%.*

Get the Facts

International Weight Trends

International Overweight and Obese Data:

- 128 countries reviewed were "overweight"
- 123 countries reviewed were "obese"
- 1 in 9 adults were obese in 2008—1 in 3 overweight
- 1 in 5 women are obese in 117 countries
- 1 in 5 men are obese in 73 countries

BEING OVERWEIGHT INCREASED DIABETES RISK

For every two pounds of added body weight, there is a 9% increased risk of diabetes.

*Sugar is not the **only issue**: I am not saying that consuming sugar is the sole culprit, but **EXCESS** sugar intake (mainly sugar drinks) is certainly a **main** contributor to the prevalence of overweight and obesity.*

What does that mean? Excess of anything, whether it is sugar, or protein, or fat, or carbs that turn to sugar, will be stored as fat if we do not use them for energy. The thing about sugar is that *foods* that **contain sugar** tend to be less filling, have zero fiber, come packed with extra calories and end up *contributing* 20% or more of **EXTRA** calories that you might **NOT**

Even 16 ounces of sugar drinks × 6 days will give you at least 12 cups of sugar beverage intake. How much sugar is that? How many extra calories could that be? If each soda has 8 to 12 teaspoons of sugar, we end up with at least 96 teaspoons of sugar per week! How about all the extra work for your pancreas and kidneys!

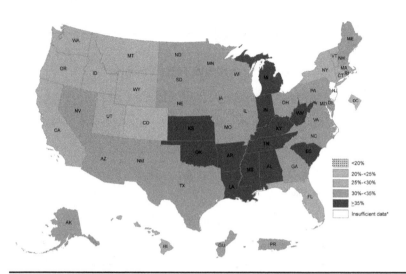

Figure 6: *Adopted from the latest CDC obesity prevalence map of 2020, you can see the darker states which suffer from increased obesity within its population. Are you part of these states? How does your culture or environment influence what you eat? Can you make some changes?* https://www.cdc.gov/obesity/data/prevalence-maps.html.

use. What is the result? Well, the extra stuff will have to be stored as fat . . . Over time, you will wonder why you gained these extra 5, 10, 20 pounds. We are seeing this in younger kids, especially my adolescent patients whose intake of high sugar drinks has surprised even me. Once I read their labs and measured their waists and saw their food and drink intake history, oh my! They consumed up to 2,000 extra calories from sugar drinks per week.

Once my patients reduce their sugar intake, remember that includes all the foods that turn to blood sugar quickly (white flour, refined flour products, cereals, sugary drinks, soda, processed food and high fructose corn syrup products), they are more likely to lose weight and keep it off more easily, as well as control blood sugar and thereby cravings.

The Ever-Increasing Diabetes Trend

Obesity is directly linked to an increased risk of diabetes, *which currently affects at least 25.8 million people in the U.S.*[40] The prevalence of diabetes in the U.S. from 1958 to 1994 increased 5-fold and approximately 5.9 million were undiagnosed. Not only does diabetes create a financial burden and is emotionally taxing, it's also the leading cause of kidney failure, nonaccident-related lower limb amputations and blindness.

Worldwide: Diabetes affects over 340 million people

United States: 35% of adults over age 20 and 50% over 65 are prediabetic

Since the dawn of the Industrial Revolution, with the invention of electronics, appliances and cars our energy output (the calories we burn per day) has decreased significantly. Most people in the Western world do not work on the farm plowing and digging for eight hours a day or washing laundry in the river for hours at a time or scrubbing floors on hands in knees. Today, people drive everywhere, sit for hours watching TV, work on computers for hours on end and have all kinds of wonderful appliances such as washing machines, dryers, dishwashers and even automatic dust picker-uppers (vacuums)! As a result, these innovations keep us sitting on our booties without moving as much as our bodies need to burn energy.

With the increased availability and abundance of foods, especially refined, processed foods and fast foods, our intake is seriously exceeding energy output. The quality of what is eaten is also not so great. Eating more of something healthy is quite different from eating more of something "junky". Consumption of processed foods with low fiber or no fiber, with added corn syrup and sugars, means added calories will not be burned. This causes an input/output imbalance which is associated with obesity and health risks including: hypertension, diabetes, osteoporosis, depression and cardiovascular disease, loss of productivity, loss of work and a lower quality of life.

Even if genetics make you prone to being curvier and larger, it is still important to reach **your healthiest, leanest** condition possible. That is why I am passionate about sharing with you the best way to find health-filled success through *Your Health, Your Body, Your Life*. Your goal is to create a balance between what you put in your body and what you burn and to become aware of how you feel with what you eat! Help decrease your health risks and increase health benefits by doing the following:

- Don't punish yourself!
- Never feel guilty!
- Enjoy food, glorious food!
- Eat when you are hungry, not when you're not!
- Learn what it *feels* like to feel satisfied and full instead of over-stuffed!
- Find fabulous activities to keep your heart pumping and muscles flexible!

Food and Calorie Trends

Do you like dining out? I love it. Who doesn't? However, if you are not careful, going out to eat can result in higher-calorie foods and larger portions! There is an increased trend in modern, fast-paced society of going out to eat. In data collected from 1994–1996, 32% of those surveyed went out to eat, which was 18% higher than in the 1970s.[41] While reviewing USDA statistics on food intake in the United States, I found that the U.S. intake of fat, sodium and sugar were much higher than recommended, with annual

Get the Facts

Fun Facts About How Much We Eat

How many pounds of red meat, poultry and fish do you think the average American consumes each year?

According to the US Department of Agriculture, current total meat consumption is 195 pounds per person per year! During the 1950's, the average intake of animal protein was a mere 57 pounds per person. Fast foods and "All You Can Eat" buffets are another culprit in the psychological battle of getting the most food for your money. But these eating-to-excess supersized meals cause you to forget to only eat what fits in your stomach rather than consuming what fits in a warehouse! The good news is you can reframe your thinking about food and money. In the long run, you will be losing money by paying for the health consequences of overeating.

consumption of 85 pounds of fat (butter, oil) and 141 pounds of sweeteners. What about fruits and veggies? Intake was extremely low, less than one serving of each per day. Curiously, an estimated intake of vegetables was calculated totaling 415 pounds per year. However, it was mainly from potatoes and corn, the sugary and starchy, bread-like version and not much of the healthy greens! For example, the average intake of sodium for adults was over 3,400 milligrams per day, while the recommended maximum is

2,200 milligrams with a healthier range between 1,500 to 2000 milligrams. Dairy intake was very high, but calcium and iron were surprisingly low (15 milligrams instead of 18 milligrams) with calcium averaging about 900 milligrams. instead of 1,200 milligrams. Of course, good old *fiber* only made it to 15 grams per day instead of the 30–45 grams that our bodies need. Here are some examples of fiber content: Medium apple 4 grams; ½ cup, cooked spinach 7 grams; ¾ cup cooked broccoli 7 grams; 1cup blackberries 9.8 grams.

EAT 'EM and FEEL GOOD: minerals, vitamins, fiber from fresh produce, nuts, seeds and more!

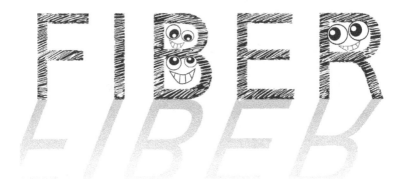

Is the American diet designed for disease? Well, sadly, the answer is **YES!** How can we change or even reverse this trend? By consuming food sources of vitamins, minerals and phytonutrients and reducing calories, fat, refined carbohydrates and animal protein. Not only healthier food, but regular exercise and adequate rest are important in decreasing disease.

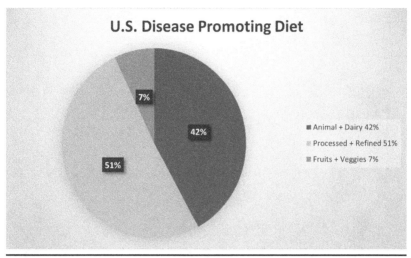

Figure 9: *Adopted from USDA Agriculture Fact Book 98: Chapter 1-A.*

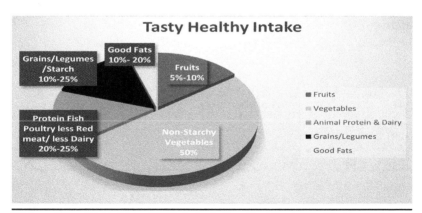

Figure 10: *Adopted from USDA Agriculture Fact Book 98: Chapter 1-A.*

What you want to eat looks more like this:

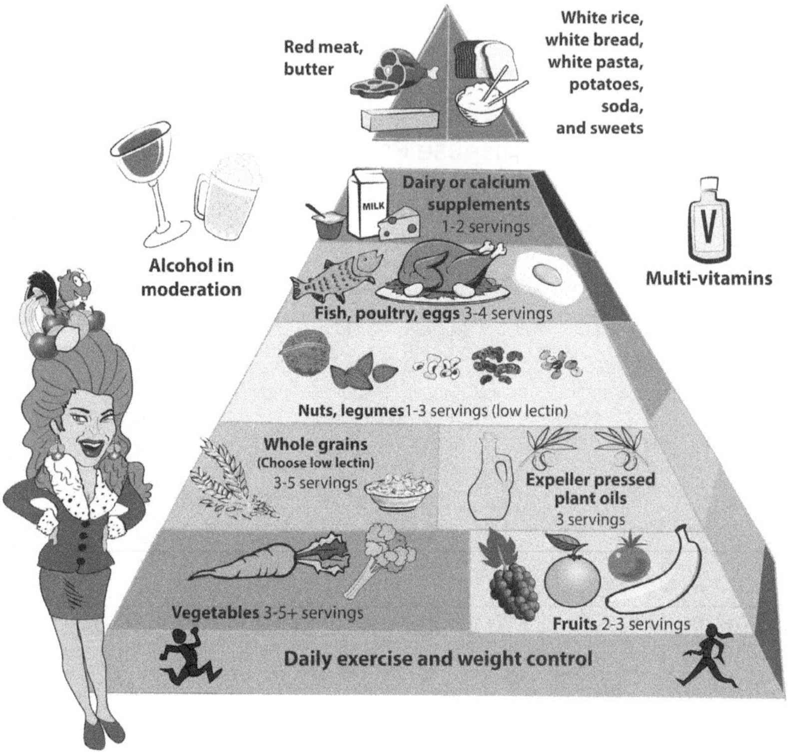

Figure 7: *Example of Health Promoting Foods by Dr. Dani, Ph.D. recommendations adopted from Harvard School of Public Health Food Pyramid Recommendations and Mediterranean Diet.*

Due to high lectin content in legumes, you can skip them, or cook them in high heat (test it)—though lectin is not totally removed this way.

Dairy can be irritating, try goat dairy or unsweetened Nut milks—you choose.

*You can substitute grain servings with small amounts of quinoa, lentils, or yams if you wish. The most effective blood sugar control and weight maintenance is seen with the lowest starchy carbohydrate and grain intake.

What are we really eating?

U.S. Population: refined grain and flour per person, annually

Most bread and cracker products in the grocery store are low in fiber and loaded with added sweeteners and fillers. Just because the label says, "wheat" or "whole wheat" does not mean you are getting the *actual whole grain* that is healthy. When it comes to healthier whole grains, only 7% of us consume the recommended 3-5 servings per day of real, unadulterated sprouted grain and whole grain (not refined and with no added bleach.)

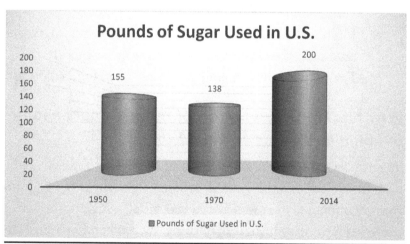

Figure 8: *Pounds of sugar consumed per person in the U.S. 1950, 155 pounds; 1970, 138 pounds; 2014, 200 pounds.*

READ THE LABEL: It was not until 1990 that the Nutrition Labeling and Education Act required food manufacturers to list ingredients and nutrition facts. Not only does it help to read the label, but you'll also want to be aware of the ingredients and what they mean. In 2010, the Affordable Care Act required restaurants, cafeterias, trains, airplanes and bakeries to label calorie and nutrition in foods. *However, it is not really making a difference in the big picture, obesity and junk food intake is still on the rise in the U.S.*

and in the world. On an individual basis, it can be very useful. If
you want to try to pay attention to label reading, here is what you
want to look for on the label of breads if you choose to eat grains:
  ✓ Organic Sprouted grain
  ✓ No sugar added
  ✓ 3 grams fiber or more
  ✓ 15-17 grams (or less) carbohydrates per slice
  ✓ Avoid fillers that contain chemical softeners or petro-
    leum derivatives

Reading the label on a package of "whole wheat crackers" I found
that there was:
  ✓ < 1 gram of fiber
  ✓ High-fructose corn syrup (sugar) and/or artificial sweet-
    eners, glucose syrup and molasses (4 sugar types)
  ✓ Foam-type fillers, chemical softeners and food coloring

Why has the consumption of refined flours nearly doubled in the last 40 years?

This is partly due to the USDA, which advocated following (the
now discarded) Food Pyramid, where large amounts of grains
were recommended, as well as the fear of fat, which pushed people to eat more carbohydrates. Fortunately, the Food Pyramid has
been revised as experts have worked to better understand what our
bodies need to be fit and healthy. Reduced grains and increased
vegetable recommendations can be found in the Harvard School
of Public Health's Healthy Eating Pyramid (see Chart.) This
chart is filled with pictures of tennis shoes and weights, someone
weighing (self-monitoring) and a drawing of a balanced plate
filled with lean protein, a small portion of wild rice and vegetables
with a glass of milk. Only a very small portion of this new pyramid has whole grains and it has generous portions of vegetables,
some fruits and good oils. (example: olive oil, walnuts). Take a

peek and discover how you can still be a happy foodie by knowing how to balance your delicious plate!

SAY CHEESE!

1950–2000: Cheese consumption increased from 7.7 pounds to 29.8 pounds per person.

That's up a whopping 287%!

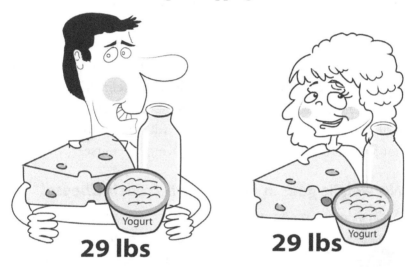

29 lbs   **29 lbs**

Some American cheeses are not traditionally fermented like slow-aged European cheeses. They are often made with oil and milk and added to processed foods such as Frozen cheese snacks like nachos, tacos, pizzas, spreads, etc. The creamy texture of cheese is addicting and contributes to a cycle of high fat intake, which can block self-regulating appetite mechanisms. It is okay to eat some cheese, as witnessed through cheese studies in France that demonstrate healthier population in France than in the U.S. and Britain, even with their high cheese intakes.[42]

Not only do Americans consume vast amounts of cheese, but a majority of America consumes processed oils, fast foods and does not eat enough vegetables/produce or nuts. Americans don't walk as much as Europeans do and frankly, there may be a positive link between French people eating aged fresh cheeses and drinking wine vs. the U.S. population drinking soda and cheese singles at a fast-food restaurant. You can measure the fat intake in total grams ingested, but really, as you can imagine, the quality of fat does matter—is it hydrogenated or is it real.

This is known as the French Paradox and many researchers have been trying to figure out why the French, with their delicious high fat brie intake, their cigarettes and their alcohol intake still have lower heart disease rates than other countries, such as Spain or Portugal, which have lower saturated fat intake. The type of fat is important to the quality of life. Most definitely, those who consume higher processed fats and junk food usually don't fare as well as those who eat real food, even if it's delicious French brie; not found at McDonald's or Burger King, of course.[43]

No weight gain in France with French Cheese!

An article by an adventurous freelance food writer published in

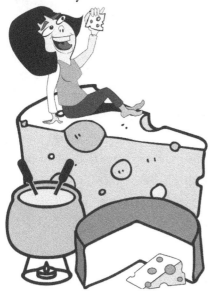

the *Huffington Post* put the French diet to the test.[44] The author traveled to Paris and decided to eat like the French. She worried she would gain weight if she didn't go to the gym after eating all that delicious French cheese, wine and chocolate. Instead of going to the gym, she found herself having fun with friends walking to cafes to indulge in decadent French food, climbing the Eiffel Tower, bike riding across the city, rowing in the lake and even going from tasty bakeries to delicious bistros—not by car, but on foot! And while she expected her skinny jeans not to zip by the end of her trip, she was pleasantly surprised that she still fit into them after a fabulous French adventure.

"French women don't *work out*". . . they eat well and have fun by staying physically active and *enjoying* being foodies. So, the question is, would you have taken the elevator or climbed the Eiffel Tower!? The concept of "working out" going to the gym is not necessary as long as your lifestyle is full of lots of physical activity. Rowing on the river and walking up the Eiffel Tower happily took the place of going to the gym for Miss McMahan!

Hold the Pepperoni . . . ! One of the health risks with pizza is pepperoni, which is filled with nitrites. Pizza eaters ate 252 million pounds of pepperoni per year! The National Cancer Institute has asked us to reduce nitrite-rich foods due to increased risk of cancer. Even at ⅛ ounce three times per week increases the risk of stomach and esophageal cancer! Americans eat about 100 acres of pizza a day; 36% topped with pepperoni. Super Bowl Sunday is the single most popular pizza day: Domino's drivers log four million miles, tips increase from $2 to $20 and delivery sales spike. The next highest pizza consumption days are New Year's Eve, Halloween, the night before Thanksgiving and New Year's Day. In the beginning of the book, I mention "cues" and "substitution behavior." Now that you are aware of these social triggers, pay attention to times you might indulge or over-consume junk food. If you do want to eat pizza, add a lot of vegetables on those days to help reduce inflammation, digestive problems and health risks. A healthier choice includes pizza with thin crust, fresh veggies and light cheese (hold the pepperoni).

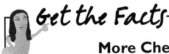

Get the Facts

More Cheesy Facts:
Pizza

$38 billion dollar industry

5 billion pizzas are sold annually world-wide

3 billion pizzas sold each year in the U.S.

Average of forty-six slices of pizza per person annually!

Americans eat so much pizza that the U.S. government launched a study of over 17,000 people (ages two and over) and found that one in eight had pizza on any given day. One in four males (ages 6–19) ate pizza every day![56]

Fun Fact Pizza Trivia:

What's the highest-grossing, single-unit independent pizzeria in the United States?

Answer: Moose's Tooth Pub and Pizza in **Alaska**!

They grossed six million dollars and Anchorage has only 300,000 people. That's a lot of pizza: it's cold up there!

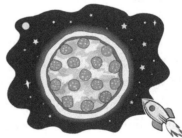

MILK

According to the USDA: dairy production in 23 states for 2013 was 16.4 billion pounds of milk.[45]

Hormones and Milk: Recent consumer preferences for "organic" or "no added hormone" milk products are part of a continual debate on the safety of drinking milk or eating meat from rBGH (a genetically engineered growth hormone called Recombinant Bovine Growth Hormone) cows. Though the FDA based its 1993 approval of rBGH on one study that lasted 90 days, performed on 30 rats, Canada's Health Canada found numerous concerns regarding the safety of rBGH. This is also true for the European Union (EU).

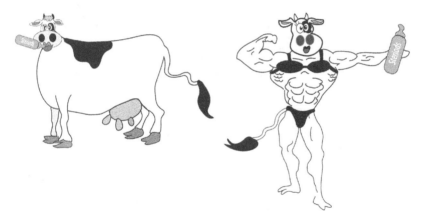

There are six other hormones including a form of estrogen called "oestrogen," which has been found to pose increased risk in developing cancer. There are three naturally occurring hormones in cows: estradiol, progesterone and testosterone and three synthetic injected hormones: zeranol, trenbolone and melengestrol. You can always choose milk products from free-range or grass-fed cows that have not been injected with synthetic hormones. Easily digestible dairy products are also available from goat and sheep's milk. However, it is interesting to note that humans are the only

Here Comes the Sun

Now we know that the sun's rays help you make important Vitamin D, but it also helps with many more things. Over 100 years ago, sun exposure was used to help tuberculosis patients. Now, it is known to help regulate melatonin, affects retina of your eye by helping biorhythms, treatment for psoriasis, dermatitis, SAD (seasonal affective disorder) and much more. Hey, plants need the sun for photosynthesis and so do we for our own form of photosynthesis, without the chlorophyll. A little doesn't mean a lot, remember, there's an increased risk of skin cancer from overexposure to sunlight. Moderation and balance are the keys.

species that drink milk from another animal after they've been weaned from their own mother's milk. How many stomachs to we have? How many stomachs do cows have? A cow's stomach has **four** compartments. Think about it. The milk from a cow is intended for a baby cow: Our digestive system is totally different: We are not cows! MOOO!

Those Who Say No

Proponents of not consuming milk at all are concerned about increased inflammation and increased risk of fractures caused by high dairy intake. Inflammation from dairy may causes skin reactions, sinus issues, digestive issues and calcium malabsorption. Curiously, the countries with the highest dairy product intake have the highest incidence of osteoporosis, such as Denmark and the U.S. However, studies do show that those having had dairy products early in life, as teens and then in post-menopausal years, have a lower risk of osteoporosis. But it's *not dose dependent*, so too much may be a problem too. Don't drink a gallon, if you drink milk, stick to your 8 ounces.

Other Calcium Sources

Remember, you can get just as much calcium from non-dairy sources, such as your dark leafy greens, sardines and salmon and even fortified milk alternatives such as Almond Milk, Rice Milk, Hemp and Flax Milk, Cashew Milk (unsweetened, without carrageenan, if possible, as it's a digestive irritant).

Dairy Issues

There is more information about these fillers in the "What's in your food" section. To the point, though not all professionals agree, there exist studies that find a correlation between higher intake of dairy and increased inflammation, as well as higher mortality and higher fractures in women.[46] Again, "confounding variables" (things that also affect something) that make it difficult to solely blame milk, but it is important to be aware. It is possible that in the case of dairy, more is not better and again, that moderation is your best friend, even with milk.

What About Calcium If I Don't Drink Milk?

How Much Calcium Do You Need?

1,000 milligrams a day is a good average and if you get enough Vitamin D, then you can absorb the calcium even better. Vitamin D is made by YOU as long as you hit a few of the sun's rays every day for at least 20 minutes, generally between 11 a.m. and 1 p.m. when the ultraviolet B (UVB) rays are most conducive to Vitamin D production in your skin. Those living in no sun environments, make sure you can get as much as you can when the sun finally does come out and ask your doctor about specific UVB lights to help you avoid the blues (in case you react to gray skies) and to help your body make Vitamin D. You get good amounts of calcium from three cups of almond milk, or one cup of Almond Milk (fortified), one cup canned salmon, two cups of turnip greens and vegetables and a cup of black-eyed peas. Get D from food and supplements.

MEATS AND PROTEIN

U.S. citizens consume 185 pounds per person per year
of chicken, turkey, pork and beef combined.

Take advantage of sales at organic markets. You can freeze free-range, organic, or grass-fed meats that are half price and use them when you are ready, instead of paying high prices. Humanely raised and organically or pasture raised farming practices, following a *5-step-animal welfare-rating-program*, as well as responsibly farmed fish options are available, if you are not vegetarian. (https://www.globalanimalpartnership.org/5-step-animal-welfare-rating-program; www.seafoodwatch.org) Processed, hormone-injected cattle, pesticide-rich and genetically or chemically modified food sources that the animals consume, as well as lack of physical mobility in modern factory farming can alter animal biochemical composition as much as it can affect you (not-withstanding ethical issues associated with some modern-day practices).

What's the Beef about added Hormones?

Apparently, a lot. Nearly 80% of U.S. feed lot cattle are injected with synthetic hormones. "Free Radical" DNA damaging effects due to oestrogen added to meat can damage DNA and affect 'oestrogen-receptor mediation' (how your receptors react). If you think of estrogen as a "key" and the receptor as the keyhole in the door that tells the cell what to do, you can imagine more clearly how added hormones impact the delicate key and door relationship in your body. Oestrogen tells your cells to keep replicating, which is the issue with cancer. Cell proliferation or uncontrolled cell replication is a description of cancer. The National Toxicology Program's Board of Counsellors, an acknowledged U.S. medical advisory panel, put the hormone Oestrogen, used in U.S. cattle raising, on the *known carcinogens* list.[47] Simply put, if DNA is altered, cancer risk increases. Humans are sensitive biochemical creatures. Altering the biochemistry has proven risky both to animals and to humans in scientific studies where DNA alterations have been confirmed.

Though 2020 and 2021 announced some gradual imports of US beef to the European Union, in 2014 the EU had banned importing US raised beef that had been treated with hormones. *The European Union (EU) has banned importing U.S. raised beef that has been treated with hormones.* Since 1985, when Europe banned the use of growth hormones in meat, U.S. meat exports to Europe dropped from 6,975 metric tons in 1997 to 106 metric tons. While this may seem like an economic nightmare for the cattle industry, the 15-country EU follows "precautionary principles". The EU has expanded their concern for human, animal and environment welfare where synthetic hormones are a concern. Europe's position states it does not want to continue unsustainable practices at any risk to human health. Here is an excerpt from an international agricultural and political journal regarding the import of U.S. hormone-treated beef:

. . . Irish Farmers' Association President John Bryan welcomed the new rule but said his group "remains resolute" on maintaining European standards in the trade deal. The European Union currently bans the import of hormone-treated beef and has a comprehensive domestic system for tracing the origins of its beef. "Neither European producers nor consumers will tolerate lower standards on traceability, the use of hormones or animal welfare," Bryan said in a news release. "EU negotiators who are engaged in talks with the U.S. side on a trade deal must keep this at the forefront of their position."[48]

As of May 2014, Germany banned the import of U.S. commercially farmed chicken. However, though chicken farming does not add hormones, U.S. commercially farmed chickens are raised with antibiotics and feed that is genetically modified and high in pesticides, and washed with chlorine, is of concern to EU, though denied by Purdue farms. (reference https://www.japantimes.co.jp /news/2020/01/28/business/u-s-wants-end-eu-ban-chlorinated -chicken-hormone-treated-beef/). Due to overcrowding, inhumane beak cutting is common. These chickens experience higher infection rates which further promotes the use of antibiotics. It is important to pay attention to current health trends and listen to concerned citizens throughout the world to increase awareness and make your own informed choices. To ensure you and your family are safe— why not eat the cleanest, least altered food possible within your means?

A first step for great health is to reduce sugars. The second wonderful step is to add high amounts of multicolored vegetables and smaller amounts of deliciously juicy fruits to help keep you healthy. (See organic and grass-fed farms and resources in chapter 6). That brings us to the idea of grass-fed, or no added-hormone meats.

Grass-fed or no-added hormone meats are also a source of debate. Animal study results regarding hormone additives have research scientists concerned about potential long-term health effects. One major effect is decreased fertility in young males.[49] While long-term studies on humans do not exist, animal studies show concerning results. The cause and effect are hard to calculate. Why? There are multiple dynamics that affect health and finding a direct link is hard to verify. Although added hormones are legal in the U.S., long-term health effects are a concern.[50,51] Many countries err on the side of caution and ban added hormones. You can read more of this in chapter six.

ALCOHOL

If you must imbibe, do so in moderation!

If you drink mixed alcoholic drinks, sweet juice and soda combinations may get you into "belly fat" trouble.[52] Don't be fooled by thinking that using diet soda in your cocktail is any better: It's actually worse, as it seems to increase the effect of the alcohol resulting in hangovers the next morning. The more you drink, the more calories you take in, so a balanced diet along with consistent physical activity helps curb fat storage from alcohol consumption. In addition, research has shown that alcohol decreases an enzyme needed to fight cancer. Beer contains fructose which not only causes a "beer belly" but also contributes to inflammation. To decrease uric acid inflammatory risks from fructose, you will want to drink fewer beers and lagers. You can consume moderate amounts of wine (one or two four-ounces glasses per day). Red wine is filled with antioxidants like resveratrol, found in fresh grapes. Studies of resveratrol (from grape skin) show beneficial effects on cholesterol through preventing the oxidizing of bad (LDL) cholesterol which forms plaque. In fact, it may help to fight off the negative consequences of increased fructose intake. Recent studies also demonstrate benefits not only from red wine, but from white wine. Remember, you can get resveratrol benefits from actual grape skin and berries, so you don't need to drink wine, but if you do, moderation is the key! Studies show that *more* than two glasses of red wine can have the opposite health effects, cancelling the beneficial effects of moderate amounts by increasing heart, blood pressure and liver health risks.

Sulfites in wine, an added preservative, above the naturally occurring sulfites from fermentation, may cause headaches and inflammatory responses in certain people. Many Italian and French wines tend to use less added sulfites. In some countries added sulfites are not allowed (try organic wines with no added sulfites).

Alcohol and Cancer Risk

According to the National Cancer Institute (NCI), regular alcohol intake increases the risk of developing cancers of the throat, voice box, esophagus, liver, breast, colon and rectum. The risk increases in those that drink alcohol and are tobacco users. How much alcohol are they talking about?! Approximately 3.5 drinks or more per day or several times per week increases the risk significantly.[53] The National Toxicology Program of the U.S. Department of Health and Human Services states that the cancer risk from alcohol is dose dependent. The more a person drinks, the higher the risk. In the U.S. about 3.5% of cancer deaths are related to alcohol. But it tastes so good! So, what do we do? Moderation is the key! Yay! As with anything, being responsible and listening to our bodies gives you the power over uncertainties.

What is moderate drinking, then? U.S. guidelines consider moderate drinking as one drink for women per day and up to two drinks for men. Heavy drinking is considered three drinks or more per day, or more than seven drinks per week for women and more than 14 drinks per week for men.

One serving of alcohol (one of these):
- 12 ounces of beer
- 8 ounces of malt liquor
- 5 ounces of wine
- 1.5 ounces ("shot") of 80-proof liquor

Cancer risks from alcohol
Head and neck cancer:
- two to three times greater risk than non-drinkers

Esophageal cancer:
- higher in those who are missing an enzyme for alcohol metabolism, higher overall than in non-drinkers
- higher for those with acid reflux

Liver cancer:
- drinking is an independent risk factor for liver cancer

Breast cancer:
- 1.5 greater risk than nondrinkers; for each 10 grams increase in alcohol (less than one drink), a 7% increased cancer risk

Colorectal cancer:
- 1.5 greater risk than non-drinkers if drink 50 grams or more

For every 10 grams of alcohol consumed, there was a 7% increase in colorectal cancer

Curiously, some alcohol intake decreased the risk of renal cancer and non-Hodgkin lymphoma (NHL), with a 15% reduction in risk of NHL. It is recommended that the _one drink rule_ applies as protective, though the mechanism of protection is not understood. Unfortunately, for smokers, all cancer risks increase, especially with alcohol intake at greater amounts.

How does alcohol affect our cells?

When alcohol breaks down, it converts into a toxic byproduct called, _acetaldehyde_, which can damage our DNA and building proteins. It also creates free radicals (reactive oxygen species) which damage cells. In addition, alcohol decreases

Cancer Risk

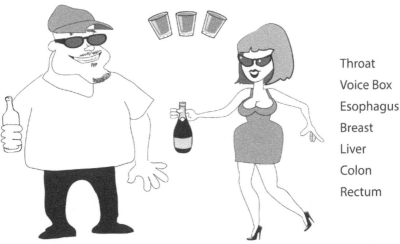

Throat

Voice Box

Esophagus

Breast

Liver

Colon

Rectum

the body's capacity to use certain nutrients vital to cellular function. Vitamin A, all B vitamins, vitamin C, vitamin D, vitamin E and the carotenoids are affected. If it's not the alcohol, then it's the added chemicals used in the production of popular alcoholic beverages. Asbestos fibers, phenols, hydrocarbons, nitrosamines and sulfites can be found in alcoholic beverages. Always use in moderation, per the National Cancer Institute's recommendations.

FAST FOOD TRENDS

How much do you love getting a juicy burger and a soda . . . or a milkshake, fries and dessert, without ever needing to get out of the car!?

When it comes to fast food junkies, I can tell my fast-food loving patients don't know what they are putting into their precious bodies. They are succumbing to cravings. Most of us have done the same thing, but it's good to recognize what we are putting in our body and how fast foods metabolize. According to the Centers for Disease Control adults consume about twelve percent of their total calories from fast food and more than ⅓ of youth aged 2–19 eat fast-food on any given day.[54] That's rough on your digestive system because your body has to process preservatives, low quality hydrogenated oils, excess sodium and heavy doses of nitrites, which the American Cancer Association associates with disease. Nitrites are associated with cancer of the esophagus and stomach. If you insist on giving in to your *cravings* of fast foods, choose healthier, nitrite-free options.

PERCENT FAST FOOD CONSUMPTION
MEN 12% AND WOMEN 11%

With age, comes wisdom. For those 60 years old or older, fast food intake comprises only 6% of the daily calories, but younger people ages 20 to 39 consume over 50% of their calories form fast

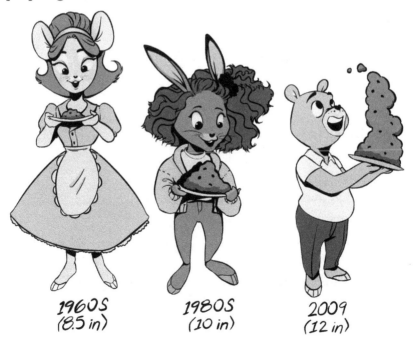

1960S
(8.5 in)   1980S
(10 in)   2009
(12 in)

food. Income does not seem to affect fast food consumption as a whole, except for in people ages 20 to 39, where lower income is associated with more fast-food intake. In my experience, over 50% of my patients (especially men—high school and college age students) eat fast food and more than 60% consume sugar drinks several times per week, with still others drinking sweet drinks at least once a day.

What we used to eat 20 years ago . . . vs. what an acutal serving is!

No matter what level of income, selecting and enjoying healthier foods can be affordable and delicious! Pay attention to portion control. **Good News**: High-fiber, healthier foods make you feel fuller, keep you full longer and keep you from "crashing" from low blood sugar. You even save money! It's true that certain healthy foods are more expensive, but if you are on a budget, try local farmers' markets, church food banks and food assistance programs (a government program now allows only fruits and vegetables to be used with the voucher). Substituting soda or non-nutritious foods with nutritious drinks can save you in the long

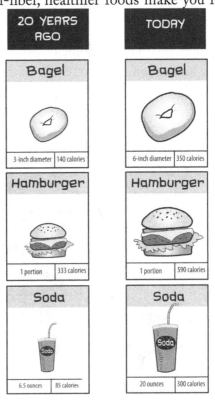

What we used to eat 20 years ago and what an acutal serving is

run by lowering potential medical bills created by obesity and diabetes risk. Spend $10 every 10 days on a soda (or even bubbly water) or on food that improves your health? No brainer! You can also make your dollar stretch by cooking eggs, dried lentils and vegetables like onions, celery and carrots with brown rice. All are inexpensive and fill you up with the added bonus of getting half of your daily fiber (15 grams of the 30 grams) in one meal!

CARBONATED SODA

Beverages with added sugar make up 22% of the added refined sugar intake of the American food supply. In 1970, carbonated soda intake and its sugar made up about 16% of the American food supply. According to Gallup, of 2,027 people surveyed, 32% drank regular soda and 24% drank diet soda. Age was a factor with 50% of those ages eighteen to twenty-nine years-old consuming sodas. In 2012, a Gallup poll found that more than 50% of all Americans consume at least one glass of soda per day.

Which country consumes the most soda? As of the end of 2019, Mexico beats us all, but only by a small margin, as the USA takes a second lead, followed by Brazil. Mexico is reported to consume 680 8-ounce servings per year per person, while the US loves its 618 8-ounce servings per person per year. Check out Statistica websites (www.statistica.com) to stay up to date.

Annual Soda Consumption per Capita (liters) vs GDP per capita 2018

- The U.S.A. has the highest global soda consumption at over 160 liters per capita per year, with a per capita GDP of $50,000 per year with its $45 billion industry.
- The average per capita consumption was 167.5 liters in 2018. According to the CDC (2020), recent data shows a hopeful reduction to 38.87 gallons per person,

Get the Facts

Side Effects of SODA

See no Evil, Hear no Evil, Speak no Evil, Drink no Evil

- Two-Fold Effect—decline in kidney function and increase in kidney failure
- Tooth Enamel Decay—Soda has acid pH of 3.2; water has a neutral pH of 7.0
- Weight Gain—thirty-four percent increase in Metabolic Syndrome (belly fat, high cholesterol)
- Increased Waistline—500% (six times more) increase than non-diet soda drinkers
- Increased Appetite (body doesn't recognize diet drink is not sugar): aspartame confuses the brain and chemical reactions can lead to headaches
- Diabetes or Blood Sugar Spikes—decrease insulin sensitivity
- Calcium Depletion from Bones—increases risk of osteoporosis. To maintain the proper pH in your blood after soda intake, calcium is removed from your bones and moved to your blood to create a less acid environment in the blood
- Digestive Problems—deteriorates stomach lining
- Increased Hangover—mixing drinks and diet soda (absorbs faster)
- DNA Damage—hives, asthma to due to mold inhibitor (sodium benzoate)

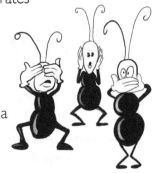

compared to its height in 2000 of 53 gallons per person. Over 30% of the population drinks daily sugar drinks, contributing to obesity.

- The average revenue per person for Soft Drinks amounted to $226.35 in 2018, but it has increased in 2020.
- Soft drink volume is expected to amount to 81,430.8 million liters (21511.74 million gallons) by 2021.
- Soft drink leaders are Coca-Cola, PepsiCo and Keurig's Dr. Pepper.

Is Diet Soda a better alternative?

Sadly, people who consume diet soda weigh considerably more than those who do not consume any type of soda. On average, of those who are overweight: 32% say they drink soda, whereas of people who fall into the healthy weight category, only 19% say they drink soda. While adult intake of sugar drinks has increased over the past decade by 25%, the startling reality is that children's intake of diet soda has *doubled*.

Okay, so does this mean regular soda is better for you than diet beverages?

Although some experts say it is okay to have one soda every now and then, the truth is, it is never advisable. Why would you want to put such a tough-to-process liquid into your body? The minute you drink a sugary soda, you have an unhealthy and inflammatory glucose rush, a spike of insulin and compensatory reactions by your body to balance pH. The soda irritates your digestive tract. In addition to consuming too much phosphorus, which leaches calcium from your bones to maintain the necessary pH level and the cumulative effects are toxic. The 12 teaspoons of sugar or corn syrup in *each* serving of soda stresses the Islets of Langerhans.

What's that you are probably asking? These form a "little town" of one million Islets in your pancreas that produce insulin in response to sugar influxes in your bloodstream.

The insulin secreted lowers your blood glucose after soda intake spikes your sugar. After this sugar spike, a load of insulin is produced and drops your sugar concentration. The result? You get a crash that makes you feel hungry and fatigued. Chronic and repeated intake of high fructose corn syrup and sugars in soda can also increase your risk of diabetes. If you insist on consuming soda, pay attention to how you *feel* afterwards (hunger, brain fog, increased cravings, nausea, bloating) and make choices that promote your goals of optimal health, energy and vitality. Some experts suggest a few sips to get rid of the craving but, be sure you have eaten first, so you are not trying to get "full" by drinking soda. In my opinion, it is best to avoid soda altogether.

Why not try black or green tea to get the caffeine fix you crave . . . ?

There are many websites that offer discounts on organic teas and foods. How about plain old water? In fact, our bodies need six to eight glasses of water per day. Actually, we need half of our body weight in ounces of water each day. For instance, if you weigh 160 pounds you need 80 ounces of water. Add more if you sweat a lot, it's hot that day, or you are exercising. See how drinking water every day works for you! If you need a little flavor, add mint leaves (for people without acid reflux "GERD"), lime, lemon, or orange slices. I like drinking filtered water, mineral water and green tea throughout the day. Green tea is full of antioxidants. I recommend organic teas to avoid excess pesticide intake from commercially grown teas.

**Try these tasty refreshing thirst quenchers
as a Soda Alternative!**

Herbal teas, Jasmine or Green teas, Water with lime, lemon, and cucumbers.

There are delicious sparkling mineral waters. Try these and feel refreshed!

CHAPTER 10

FODMAPS!

Time to take care of your Intestines
BEWARE OF FODMAP
(If you have tummy problems)

What Are FODMAPs?

THESE FOODS ARE not digestible to some people and create extreme bloating and pain.

Low FODMAP! What's that? For those suffering with irritable bowel syndrome (IBS) or Crohn's Disease, the horrible intestinal inflammation and reactivity of the colon can make life unbearable, often so debilitating, that you cannot leave the house.

FODMAPs are Fructo-oligo and di-saccharides that are not broken down properly found in high fiber and gluten products, as well as in many fruits, vegetables and beans. These cause a hot mess in those suffering with intestinal issues.

Recently, I saw a man suffering from horrible IBS/Crohn's disease, "I go to the bathroom over 50 times per day, I live on the toilet, I can't take it anymore. My doctor said that's just the way it is." Mr. X was so distraught. I gave him a low FODMAP food list, told him to write a food intake symptom journal and advised him to begin taking probiotics. One month later, I found a thank you note on my desk. "Thank you. The low FODMAP diet has made an incredible difference." On our follow-up appointment he explained, "I am able to go outside more and I only use the bathroom less than 10 times per day mostly, I think the probiotics are helping too."

> ## FODMAP: Here is what each letter means
>
> **Fermentable**
>
> (Fermented undigestible carbohydrates that cause bloating and discomfort, diarrhea, or constipation)
>
> **Oligosaccharide**
>
> (Fructans/GOS means galacto-oligosaccharides)
>
> (a prebiotic that ferments—in certain grains and foods, onions/garlic, wheat and Rye, beans)
>
> **Disaccharide**
>
> (di means 2 chains) (Lactose in Dairy cheese, yogurts)
>
> **Monosaccharide**
>
> (1 chain) Fructose in honey, fruits, corn syrup)
>
> and
>
> **Polyols**
>
> (mannitol, sorbitol and in some fruits/veggies sugar alcohols)

There are incredible resources online from universities and organizations that offer recipe ideas and food lists. For a brief overview, I am giving you a quick peek list so that you have a reference idea in case you or your loved ones need a little help in this matter.

Keeping a food journal and symptom log will help you and your loved one, figure out which foods help to decrease and which food exacerbate the IBS symptoms. You are you best teacher! Try to avoid food high in FODMAPs as the gut irritation will get worse. Give it a try. It's also good to include probiotics (acidophilus strains etc.), but not prebiotics! Prebiotics have fermentable fibers that are worse for IBS and Crohn's disease, even though they are good for those without Crohn's or IBS. Probiotics come in capsules and liquid and exist in fermented foods.

FODMAP TO DO and *NOT TO DO*
for IBS/Crohn's disease sufferers

High FODMAP	Low FODMAP
Do Not Do	**Give It A Try!**
Veggies and Bean/Legumes to avoid	Veggies and Beans/Legumes you may try
Beans Garlic/Onions/Shallots/ Scallions/Leek Cauliflower Celery High fiber vegetables Mushrooms Mixed vegetables Peas Taro Whole Grains	Broccoli Butternut squash Collard Greens Cucumber Green Beans Lentils Leek leaves (not bulb) Potatoes Squash Yam Zucchini
FRUITS to avoid	**FRUITS you may try**
Apples Avocado Blackberries Grapefruit Lychee Pears Watermelon	Bananas Blueberries Grapes Kiwi Lemon/Lime Orange Pineapple
Grains and Nuts to avoid	**Grains and Nuts you may try**
Almond meal Cashews Couscous Gluten wheat products Granola Spelt Rye	Buckwheat Corn flour Gluten free without fructose Gnocchi Hazelnut Oat (for some) not bread Rice

Dairy to avoid	Dairy you may try
Buttermilk and milk Cheese: cream, ricotta, cream Ice cream and gelato Sour cream and yoghurt	Butter Brie, Cheddar, cottage, feta, goat *chevre*, mozzarella, Swiss, Parmesan Lactose free yogurt (try)
PROTEIN, okay	PROTEIN, okay

Get the Facts

Helpful Probiotic Strains

Here is a list of some of the hundreds of probiotics studies used in healthcare globally:

Adapted from my www.drdaniphd.com website, here are some commonly used and studied strains.

(L = Lactobacillus; B = Bifidobacterium; S = Streptococcus) (yeast source Saccharomyces boulardii)

L. Acidophilus: Protects the integrity of the intestinal wall (small intestine) and helps digestion, absorption, decreases diarrhea.

L. Rhamnosus: Improves immune function, reduces allergies, IBS symptoms, vaginosis and cholesterol metabolism; studies demonstrate less sick days in those tested who used this probiotic

L. Helveticus: Swiss studies demonstrate blood pressure reduction, sleep aid and parathyroid hormone influence with increased serum calcium, which is why it may help reduce blood pressure. It's used in Swiss cheese cultures in Europe.

L. Reuteri: Reduces H. pylori bacteria (ulcers), vaginosis/candidiasis, reduces risk of gingivitis and plaque formation, reduces inflammation processes such as pro-inflammatory cytokines, helps decrease stomach problems such as nausea and gas, reduces infant colic attacks and protects against cold/flu and has been shown to help decrease dermatitis (by improving the integrity of the intestinal wall).

L. Casei: Improves immune function, cholesterol profile, digestion, reduces allergic response and is used in food production (green olives, fermented foods and cheese/yogurt).

L. Bulgaricus: Improves lipid profiles (lowers cholesterol/triglycerides), improves digestion, decreases leaky gut syndrome, inflammation, tooth decay and diarrhea/nausea, improves dairy digestion and overall gut integrity.

L. Plantarum: Makes lysine, an essential amino acid, helpful against herpes viruses. This probiotic helps digestion, immune function and is a tough cookie which helps fight against other pathogens.

L. Salivarus: Produces its OWN ANTIBIOTIC, improves immune function and digestion. It decreases risk of caries/gingivitis, some strains of strep throat.

L. Brevis/Breve: Decreases risk of mouth ulcers, stomach ulcers related to H. pylori bacteria and reduces urinary oxalate levels (less kidney stone risk)

B. Infantis: Declines as we age as it is given to babies through mom's breast milk. It is important for digestion, reduction in bloating and constipation. It fights against parasites, pathogens and mitigates kidney stones, vaginal infection and allergies.

B. Lactis: Aids in absorptions of vitamins and minerals, improves immune function and has been scientifically shown to enhance immunity, fight tumor growth and improve digestion and lower cholesterol.

B. Bifidum: This is the most common in the body (large intestine) and it helps a plethora of physiological functions: fights against candidiasis, cholesterol, digestive problems such as diarrhea and E. coli infection.

B. Coagulans: Israel, France and Germany use this probiotic to help against pathogens and viruses as it is effective and hardy (survives stomach acid well).

Lactogg Lactobacillus Rhamnosus: Improves glucose control, adheres well to gut lining so that other probiotics can be supported, improves immune function, decrease infections (ear/respiratory), reduces inflammation (eczema), stimulates NK tumor killing activity, and reduced LDL cholesterol.

S. thermophilus: Improves digestion, increases antitumor activity, increases good cholesterol HDL (high density lipoprotein), fights Clostridium difficile, improves lactose tolerance (lactose digestion), reduces risk of kidney stone formation, reduces baby colic, improves infant probiotic flora (when not breast fed).

MICROBIOME: PREBIOTICS AND PROBIOTICS. WHAT'S THE DIFFERENCE?

Just like it sounds, **Prebiotic** ("pre") is the fermentable fiber that **precedes** the formation of your own **Probiotics**. Yes, you can take probiotics and they come in fermented foods and cultured and aged dairy products, but you can also help make them with fiber rich plant- based foods which serve as a prebiotic.

Microbiome

The environment in which your own bacteria, viruses, fungi and single cell organisms (archaea) live is known as your microbiome: This is over 55% of your makeup! Scientists report there are almost *30 trillion* bacterial cells in our bodies with over 500 different kinds of natural flora (good bacteria) known as probiotics. Every surface of your body has its own colony of bacteria, fungi and microorganisms.

Since body functions are aided by probiotics (good bacteria) and are improved by Prebiotics (fibers that ferment to help you make probiotics), we better get on that NOW! The benefits include improved immune function, digestion, lactose tolerance, energy levels, lipid profiles (cholesterol) and improved communication between gut and brain, as well increased fat metabolism and improved biochemical functions.

What does it have to do with weight? There are several studies demonstrating the benefits of probiotics in obesity management, digestion and immune function. When there is a deficiency of certain probiotics, an imbalance in the microbiome results in increased risk of obesity and health problems can occur. It's important to build your natural gut flora!

Sources of Prebiotics

Raw garlic, raw or cooked onion, raw leeks, dandelion greens, raw jicama, raw asparagus, cabbage, Brussel's sprouts, broccoli, cauliflower, kale, collard greens, radish, rutabaga, raw chicory root, acacia gum (gum arabica)

Sources of Probiotics

Fermented foods (not vinegar processing) such as sauerkraut, kombucha, sourdough, kimchi and aged or fermented dairy such as yogurt, cottage cheese and Swiss cheese. They can also be taken as supplements.

Probiotics: What Do They Do?

Probiotics are food for Your Tummy, Brain, Cardiovascular System, Immune System and More!

The most common probiotic, Lactobacillus acidophilus, was discovered by Nobel Prize winner, Llya Metchnikov, in the 1890s, after having discovered L. Bulgaricus in 1882 and now, it is touted in commercials and available through hundreds of supplement companies.

Since then, 100s of strains have been identified and each decade new and marvelous discoveries are made confirming the physiological functions and benefits of a healthy multiorganism colony of "probiotics" in your body: microbiome

Not all supplements are created equal. (**Helpful Probiotic Strains Follows**)

WHY THE GUT?

This is all about your **GUT—BRAIN CONNECTION**—make sure you remember you are not made up of separate compartments but that all these compartments are interconnected—these include not only your physical state and function, but your emotional state and function.

IT'S ALL ABOUT YOU!

Eating food sources that come from the Earth vs. a factory (made up in a lab), will change your life.

> **Note from Dr. Dani**
>
> The purpose of all this information is for you to have knowledge to adapt and adopt relevant information so you can reach your ultimate Health.
>
> **THE KEY IS BALANCE.**

Eating real food like fruits and vegetables and avoiding processed packaged sugary foods and non-nutritive foods will help you feel better. This is not just about your body, but about your **brain**, your **mood**, your **motivation**, your **belief in yourself** and all the things that keep you going.

CHOOSE HEALTH.
TRUST YOURSELF.

Anything you do is good. All your new choices are good.

What you enjoy you must continue, as life is short and you can set yourself up for health with every step and choice you make. What works for someone else, doesn't necessarily work for you. Choose what you know inherently that is healthy but good and delicious, add the tasty to the special treats and make your body happy with great plant-based foods and sprinklings of the other fun foods—dark chocolate and all the things you love. Choose the cleanest foods possible—instead of high corn syrup processed chocolates, choose treats made from real ingredients you recognize that have not been so altered—real sugar, real cocoa, real butter, fresh fruits, vegetables, nuts, seeds, organic sprouted grains, some legumes if you tolerate them, palm full of grass fed meats if you eat them and experiment with new veggies roasted and drizzled with great olive oil and onions and garlic powder so your body can process the meats you like—try 8 ounces instead of 32 and reduce as you listen to your body, while increasing the other stuff...fill your plate with all the colors of that rainbow—so corny, but true. Each color will do something awesome for you—the grape skin color, the orange squash, the green kiwi, the red cabbage (if you can), the red wine (more is not better!) . . . your intuition knows . . . the best thing we can all do is listen to our intuition . . . and our bodies. If you feel horrible, then you get to make the changes that inspire your health and keep those up.

YOU ARE YOUR BEST TEACHER!

Endnotes

1   Michael J Orlich, Gary E Fraser, Vegetarian diets in the Adventist Health Study 2: a review of initial published findings, *The American Journal of Clinical Nutrition*, Volume 100, Issue suppl_1, July 2014, Pages 353S–358S, https://doi.org/10.3945/ajcn.113.071233

2   Crowe, Francesca L, Paul N Appleby, Ruth C Travis, and Timothy J Key. "Risk of hospitalization or death from ischemic heart disease among British vegetarians and nonvegetarians: results from the EPIC-Oxford cohort study". *American Journal of Clinical Nutrition*, January 30, 2013 DOI: 10.3945/ajcn.112.044073

3   Shou, H., et al., "Cognitive behavioral therapy increases amygdala connectivity with the cognitive control network in both MDD and PTSD." *NeuroImage: Clinical*, 14 (2017), 464-470. doi:10.1016/j.nicl.2017.01.030

4   Laitner, Melissa H., Samantha A. Minski, and Michael G. Perri. "The role of self-monitoring in the maintenance of weight loss success." *Eating behaviors* 21 (2016): 193-197.

https://www.ncbi.nlm.nih.gov/pmc/articles/PMC6416539/

5   Baker, Raymond C., and Daniel S. Kirschenbaum. "Self-monitoring may be necessary for successful weight control." *Behavior Therapy* 24.3 (1993): 377-394..

6   Harvard Health Publishing. (n.d.). "Why people become overweight." *Harvard Health*. http://www.health.harvard.edu/newsweek/Why-people-become-overweight.htm.

7   Skeer, M. R. and E. L. Ballard. "Are Family Meals as Good for Youth as We Think They Are? A Review of the Literature on Family Meals as They Pertain to Adolescent Risk Prevention." *Journal of Youth and Adolescence*, 42 (7), (2013) 943–963. doi:10.1007/s10964-013-9963-z.

8 Breed and Moore. https://www.sciencedirect.com/topics/medicine-and-dentistry/satiety.

9 NCBI Pubmet. https://www.ncbi.nlm.nih.gov/pubmed/17212793

10 Carter, Brett E., and Adam Drewnowski. "Beverages containing soluble fiber, caffeine, and green tea catechins suppress hunger and lead to less energy consumption at the next meal." *Appetite* 59.3 (2012): 755-761..

11 Clark, M. J., and J. L. Slavin. "The effect of fiber on satiety and food intake: a systematic review." *Journal of the American College of Nutrition*, 32 (3) (2013), 200–211.

Jarrar, A. H., et al., "Effect of High Fiber Cereal Intake on Satiety and Gastrointestinal Symptoms during Ramadan. Nutrients," 11 (4), (2019) 939. And NIH: https://www.ncbi.nlm.nih.gov/pmc/articles/PMC6521042/.

12 Eijsvogels, T. M., et al., "Exercise at the extremes: the amount of exercise to reduce cardiovascular events." *Journal of the American College of Cardiology*, 67 (3), (2016) 316–329.

13 CDC. 2014. http://www.cdc.gov/diabetes/pubs/factsheet11.htm. 2011. http://www.cdc.gov/diabetes/pubs/pdf/ndfs_2011.pdf.

14 Verhoef, S., et al., "Concomitant changes in sleep duration and body weight and body composition during weight loss and 3-mo weight maintenance." *American Journal of Clinical Nutrition* 98, (2013) no. 1: 24–31.

15 Jones, KE, RK Johnson, and JR Harvey-Berino. "Is losing sleep making us obese?" *Nutrition Bulletin*, 33 (5), (2008) 272–278.

16 Higuchi, Shigekazu, et al., "Effects of playing a computer game using a bright display on presleep physiological variables, sleep latency, slow wave sleep and REM sleep." *Journal of Sleep Research*, 14 (3), (2005) 267–273.

17 Fossum, Ingrid Nesdal, et al., "The association between use of electronic media in bed before going to sleep and insomnia symptoms, daytime Sleepiness, morningness, and chronotype." *Behavioral Sleep Medicine*, 12 (5), (2014) 343–357.

18 Thomee, Sara, Annika Harenstam, and Mats Hagberg. "Mobile phone use and stress, sleep disturbances, and sumptoms of depression among young adults—a prospective cohort study." *BMC Public Health*, 11 (66) (2011).

19 Wrenn, E. *Can't tear yourself away from the computer? Too much time online can lead to stress, sleeping disorders and depression.* July 18, 2012. : http://www.dailymail.co.uk/sciencetech/article-2175230/Too-time-online-lead-stress-sleeping-disorders-depression.html#ixzz3DmGboyJ2.

20 Ibid.

21 Arora, T, S et al., "Exploring the complex pathways among specific types of technology, self-reported sleep duration and body mass index in UK adolescents." *International Journal of Obesity*, 37 (9), (2013) 1254–1260.

22 Ibid.

23 Frappier, Julie, et al. "Energy expenditure during sexual activity in young healthy couples." *PLoS one* 8.10 (2013): e79342.

24 Krabbe, K.S., et al., "Brain-derived neurotrophic factor (BDNF) and type 2 diabetes." *Diabetologia* 50, no. 2 (2007): 431–438.

Maxfield, L. This is what happens when you drink soda. March 28, 2013. http://www.ksl.com/?nid=1-1-and-sid=24552939#83TeWrZZAef1gJ5q.99.

Miltra, A., Gosnell, B.A., Schloth, H.B., Grace, M.K., Klockars, A., Olszewski, P.K., and Levine, A.S. "Chronic sugar intake dampens feeling-related activity of neurons synthesizing a satiety mediator, oxytocin." Peptides 31, no. 7 (2011): 1346–1352.

Molteni, R., Barnard, R.J., Ying, Z., Roberts, C.K., and Go-mez-Pinilla, F. "A high-fat, refined sugar diet reduces hippcampal brain-derived neurotrophic factor, neuronal plasticity, and learning." 112, no. 4 (2002): 803-814.

25 Perlmutter MD, David. *Grain Brain; the surprising truth about Wheat, Carbs, and Sugar—Your Brain's Silent Killers.* New York: Little, Brown and Company, (2013).

26 Amen, Tana. *The OMNI Diet: the revolutionary 70% plant + 30% protein program to lose weight, reverse disease, figh inflammation, and change your life forever.* New York: St. Martin's Griffin, (2013).

27 Meyer, O. "Combined chronic toxicity/carcinogenicity study with DATEM in rats.'" Unpublished report No. IT 890451 from the Institute of Toxicology, National Food Agency of Denmark

28 Keerman, Mulatibieke, et al. "Mendelian randomization study of serum uric acid levels and diabetes risk: evidence from the Dongfeng-Tongji cohort." *BMJ Open Diabetes Research and Care* 8.1 (2020): e000834.

29 Wilhelmi de Toledo, Françoise, et al. "Unravelling the health effects of fasting: A long road from obesity treatment to healthy life span increase and improved cognition." *Annals of Medicine* (2020): 1-15.

30 de Cabo, Rafael, and Mark P. Mattson. "Effects of intermittent fasting on health, aging, and disease." *New England Journal of Medicine* 381.26 (2019): 2541-2551.

31 Lara-Castro, Cristina, and W. Timothy Garvey. "Intracellular lipid accumulation in liver and muscle and the insulin resistance syndrome." *Endocrinology and metabolism clinics of North America* 37.4 (2008): 841-856. (1992).

32 Warner, M. *The New York Times Business.* (2006, February 12). Retrieved from The Lowdown on Sweet?: http://www.nytimes.com/2006/02/12/business/yourmoney/12sweet.html?pagewanted=all and_r=0.

33   Rycer, K., and J. Jaworska-Adamu. "Effects of aspartame metabolites on astrocyts and neurons." *Folia Neurophatholica/ Association of Polish Neuropathologists And Medical Research Centre, Police Academy of Sciences* 51, no. 1 (2013): 10–17.

34   American Cancer Society (ACS). Retrieved from https:// www.cancer.org/cancer/cancer-causes/aspartame.html.

35   "Courses." *Aspartame.* (2014). http://courses.bio.indiana. edu/L104-Bonner/F09/imagesF09/L6/DietCoke.html.

36   Arora, *International Journal of Obesity*, 37.

37   Ibid.

38   Schmidt, J. C., "Serum uric acid concentrations in meat eaters, fish eaters, vegetarians and vegans: a cross-sectional analysis in the EPIC—Oxford cohort." *PLoS One*, 8 (2), (2013) e56339.

39   Ornish, D., Low-carbohydrate diets. "The Spectrum: A Scientifically Proven Program to Feel Better, Live Longer, Lose Weight, Gain Health." *Annals of Internal Medicine* 141, no. 9 (2004): 738. New York: Ballantine, 2008.

40   Ibid. CDC (2014).

41   *USDA. Economic Research Service, based on information from USDA-accredited State and private organic certifiers.* USDA, n.d. *Food Consumption and Nutrient Intakes.* (2014). http://www. ers.usda.gov/data-products/food-consumption-and-nutrient-in- takes.aspx#.Uw5EtYWhYQc.

42   Law, Malcolm, and Nicholas Wald. "Why Heart Disease Mortality Is Low in France: The Time Lag Explanation." *BMJ : British Medical Journal* 318.7196 (1999) 1471–1480.

43   Blogger http://myheartsisters.org/2010/07/17/heart-dis- ease-countries/, http://www.hsph.harvard.edu/nutritionsource/ low-fat/.

44   McMahan, D. (2013, April 14). *French Women Don't Work Out.* Retrieved from Huffpost Healthy Living, http:// www.huffingtonpost.com/dana-mcmahan/french-women-exer- cise_b_3047601.html#es_share_ended.

148

45 USDA. *Milk Production.* (2013, April 19). Retrieved from USDA: http://www.usda.gov/nass/PUBS/TODAYRPT/mkpr0413.pdf.

46 Michaelsson, K., et. al., "Milk intake and risk of mortality and fractures in women and men" Cohort Studies. *BMJ,* 349, (2014) g6015.

47 FDA. *The use of steroid hormones for growth promotion in food-producing animals XVI (V).* (2002). http://www.fda.gov/AnimalVeterinary/NewsEvents/ FDAVeterinarianNewsletter/ucm110712.htm.

48 Behsudi, Adam. "Lifting European Union beef ban may aid transatlantic deal." *Politico Pro.* (November 6, 2013). http://www.politico.com/story/2013/11/us-eu-beef-ban-trade-deal-99412.html.

49 Laurence, Peter. "Trade deal eases EU-US beef war over hormones." *BBC News Europe.* (March 14, 2012).

50 Ibid.

51 Galbraith, H. "Hormones in international meat production: biological, sociological and consumer issues." *Nutrition Research Reviews* 15, no. 2 (2002): 293–314.

52 Johnson, R.J., MD, Gower, T., and Gollub, E., Phd, RD. *The Sugar Fix: High-Fructose Fallout That is Making You Fat and Sick.* New York, NY: Pocket Books, a division of Simon and Schuster, Inc., (2008).

53 NCI. *Alcohol and Cancer Risk.* (2014, May 26). Retrieved from National Cancer Institute and the National Institute of Health: http://www.cancer.gov/cancertopics/factsheet/Risk/alcohol.

54 CDC. Vikraman, M.D., M.P.H., et al., *Caloric Intake From Fast Food Among Children and Adolescents in the United States,* (2011–2012) https://www.cdc.gov/nchs/products/databriefs/db213.htm.

55 Poirier, K. L., et al., *Effect of Commercially Available Sugar-Sweetened Beverages on Subjective Appetite and Short-Term Food Intake in Boys*. Nutrients, 11(2), (2019). 270.

Bennett, L. J., et al., *Effect of Commercially Available Sugar-Sweetened Beverages on Subjective Appetite and Short-Term Food Intake in Girls*. Nutrients, 10 (4), (2018) 394. https://www.mdpi.com/2072-6643/10/4/394.

Thornhill, K., Charlton, K., Probst, Y., and Neale, E. "Does an increased intake of added sugar affect appetite in overweight or obese adults, when compared with lower intakes? A systematic review of the literature." *British Journal of Nutrition*, 121(2), (2019) 232-240. doi: https://doi.org/10.1017/S0007114518003239.

Mandel, N., and Brannon, D. "Sugar, perceived healthfulness, and satiety: When does a sugary preload lead people to eat more?" *Appetite*, 114, (2017) 338-349. https://www.sciencedirect.com/science/article/abs/pii/S0195666317305196.

56 The Week Staff. *America's pizza obsession: By the numbers*. (2011). Retrieved from The Week http://theweek.com/article/index/216550.

Meet the Author

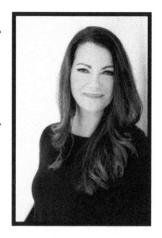

DR. M. DANIELA TORCHIA, also known as "Dr. Dani," is a professor of public health and nutrition. She has been in practice as a clinical nutritionist for over 24 years and contributes her expertise to magazines, radio, podcasts, and television. Her international background gives her a unique perspective of individual needs and the importance of adapting health counseling to the realities of her client's distinctive experiences, lifestyles, and perspectives.

Her life has been dedicated to helping others, not only in low-income clinics, but also for those struggling with their health and seeking guidance and motivation. She is an avid supporter of animal rescue organizations, national and international child sponsor programs, and aspires to contribute only what is encouraging to help make positive changes in people's lives.

Born in Europe to Austrian and Italian-American parents, she was raised in Madrid until her ninth birthday when she moved to Wheeling, West Virginia to be with her cousins. Dr. Dani remained there until her tenth birthday when she moved to Hollywood, California.

Recently, the call of Florida's tropical Gulf Coast beckoned, resulting in her cross-country journey with her husband, Tony, and their rescue tabby, Mr. Monkey where she now resides.

www.drDaniPhd.com